# Nutrition in the Nineties: Policy Issues

*Edited by*

MARGARET R. BISWAS
MAMDOUH GABR

DELHI

# OXFORD UNIVERSITY PRESS

BOMBAY  CALCUTTA  MADRAS

1994

Oxford University Press, Walton Street, Oxford OX2 6DP

Oxford  New York  Toronto
Delhi  Bombay  Calcutta  Madras  Karachi
Kuala Lumpur  Singapore  Hong Kong  Tokyo
Nairobi  Dar es Salaam  Cape Town
Melbourne  Auckland  Madrid

and associates in
Berlin  Ibadan

First published 1994

ISBN  0 19 563393 8

Printed in India
Typeset by Vibrant, Rohini, Delhi 110085
Printed at Crescent Printing Works Pvt. Ltd., New Delhi 110001
Published by Neil O'Brien, Oxford University Press
YMCA Library Building, Jai Singh Road, New Delhi 110001

This book is dedicated to
EDWARD SCHREYER
former Governor General of Canada
as a mark of esteem for a great statesman, and
a token of true regard for a friend

# Contents

# Preface

This book presents a discussion of the major policy issues with regard to nutrition and development which have been evolving during the last decade. The major issues for the nineties were arrived at in consultation with members of the IUNS Committee on Nutrition and Development. The members include some of the leading world experts on nutrition policy and planning.

This book is not in any way a duplication of *Nutrition and Development* written a decade ago. It may be considered a sequel to the earlier book, but its focus differs from it in addressing nutrition issues such as ageing, trends in diet and environment, nutrition education which are relevant to industrialized countries as well as developing countries. Its focus is not entirely on developing countries.

While the book *Nutrition and Development* is still relevant and being used, new major issues are evolving for the nineties as multitudes of rural poor migrate to overcrowded cities in search of a better life. This results in new problems for feeding the urban populace and increased pollution with consequent ill health and negative consequences for nutrition. Increasing food production to feed growing populations is contributing to deterioration of the physical environment. In Asia, the spectre of increased hunger threatens again as the man to arable land ratio decreases while high yielding varieties no longer promise continuing miracles. Africa has its own set of problems. Fortunately, there is renewed interest in solving the problem of hunger and reducing malnourishment.

Changes in food consumption due to increased affluence have resulted in chronic non-communicable diseases becoming major health problems in developing nations as well as industrialized nations. Understanding of the relationship of diet and life-style to degenerative diseases such as cardiovascular diseases, diabetes mellitus, and obesity is increasing. Most nations are also experiencing an increasing elderly population. This calls for research in geriatric nutrition.

Perhaps the major realization that emerges from the book is the need for education in general, and for nutrition and health education in particular, especially in developing countries in order to solve nutrition problems. More research is also required to establish what an ideal diet is in different cultures and ecological environments. It is not generally realized that agricultural development in industrialized countries such as the United States and Japan was accompanied by a parallel development in education that has not taken place in developing countries.

While education of women may be the main solution, the population explosion must be addressed from all angles, including religious opposition to contraception. An overcrowded world reduces the life-style of everyone whether through increased pollution, disease or perpetuation of poverty and hunger.

Although this is a policy book, it contains considerable original information as some chapters are the product of major studies. The contributors to the book are well-known in their fields with considerable experience in policy, planning, and implementation. The book is of interest to policy-makers, programme administrators, scholars, and individuals interested in nutrition policy and national development. It will also be useful as a reference text for university courses on nutrition.

In the opening chapter, Margaret Biswas discusses how modern agriculture has reduced hunger, but not without averse effects on the physical environment and on human health. Land has been degraded, water resources have been depleted, and genetic resources have been lost. There have been negative impacts on human health because of agricultural inputs. These inputs are, however, just a few of many chemical and biological contaminants of food and water. Most ill health and premature death continues to be caused by biological agents in the environment, in food, water and soil. As pointed out, many of these environmental problems have solutions, but the vast growth of populations, especially in some developing countries, renders it very difficult to implement them, and to provide adequate nutrition for all.

In Chapter 2, C. Gopalan discusses the six factors contributing to recent changes in food consumption patterns. The green revolution with emphasis on wheat and rice has resulted in indirectly contributing to a distortion of the pattern of relative availability of food grains. Improvements in the diet and health services, however, have resulted in the near elimination of florid nutritional deficiency disease. Increased urbanization in poor countries will pose the greatest challenge to nutrition in the next two decades, especially with regard to children in slums. The affluent will develop the degenerative diseases prevailing in the industrialized countries, such as coronary heart disease. In the developed countries, there are also positive developments: a return to breast-feeding, steep reduction of coronary heart diseases and a decline of certain kinds of cancer. Indian food habits continue to be cereal based but have changed. The West is also recognizing the virtue of vegetarianism. These factors provide a great chance for nutrition education.

In Chapter 3, Sarah Atkinson points out that the urban population is growing disproportionately fast, especially the poor. Also, the idea that chronic degenerative diseases will be limited to the urban elites is not factual, the poor are developing both kinds of disease patterns. Access to food and health will have to be supplied to them in the constraints of structural adjustment. Crucial issues are how to replace the demand for imported foods with local ones, and how to support the informal sector to enable it to supply increased employment and economic growth. Governments should encourage urban agriculture which has a huge production potential. Street foods viewed undesirable by governments are probably safe if eaten soon after purchase. The influence of advertising on food choice and urban pollution and food contamination are important health issues.

In Chapter 4, Mark Wahlqvist, Widjaja Lukito, and Bridget H-H.Hsu-Hage discuss, nutrition and health relationships in the aged with lessons learned from studies in the Western Pacific, Central America and IUNS studies of the elderly. Progressive ageing of populations in developing countries must be addressed. The application of rapid assessment procedures is inexpensive and an effective way of studying culturally diversified elderly populations. People of all nations with different food culture can have a comparable life expectancy and morbidity rates. It is therefore necessary to identify common foods and dietary habits which may lower mortality, for example fish in Japan, the Mediterranean and Scandinavia. Geriatric nutrition must be taught in medical schools and nutrition education in community health programmes in all countries.

In Chapter 5, Eileen Kennedy, Pauline Peters and Lawrence Haddad examine female-headed households in Africa. Since the mid-seventies, the percentage of women-headed households has been increasing in industrialized and developing countries. In the Western countries divorce and widowhood have been the major reasons, while in developing countries, rural-to-urban migration by single women in Latin America and by men in Africa has led to an increase in female-headed households. The authors examine the health and nutritional status of women and children in different household structures in Kenya, Ghana and Malawi. Female-headed households which arise as a result of traditional patterns sanctioned by society as in these countries, are less likely to be poor. This may not be true elsewhere. Data indicates women earn less than men and are less likely to have access to credit. The nutritional status of preschoolers and women cannot consistently be related to the gender of the head of household.

In Chapter 6, Mohamed El-Ghorab and Mamdouh Gabr state that nutrition education is considered unique from other types of health education because improved nutrition requires sustained and repeated change in individual behaviour. While dissemination of information through television, radio, and posters, newspapers etc. has increased knowledge of target audiences, it has had a limited effect on changing nutritional behaviour. It is most effective when used in group sessions allowing audience participation. Group discussions leading to a decision may be one of the good methods to modify social behaviour. Television, however, is not used widely enough in developing countries for education|purposes.

In Chapter 7, David Sahn discusses the effect of economic adjustment on the nutritional status of the populations of African countries. He concludes that the impact is mixed, not producing any major positive or negative changes with regard to malnutrition. The negative impacts of adjustment occur in countries like Zaire, Somalia, and Zambia which have been least committed to the process. In contrast, higher incomes, investment in social and physical infrastructure and human capital, the basis for reducing malnutrition, have occurred in countries such as Ghana, Guinea, Madagascar and Tanzania that have been deeply committed to reform. There is an increasing acceptance by countries that nutrition was harmed by conditions prior to adjustment but privatization alone will not restore growth and eliminate malnutrition.

In the final chapter, M. Amer Hussein and Wafaa Moussa in a case study of nutrition in Egypt isolate protein energy malnutrition and iron deficiency anaemia as the most prevalent types of malnutrition. Other micronutrient deficiencies such as rickets, Vitamin A, riboflavin exist but are not considered public health problems. Obesity is, however, emerging as one, while diet related diseases such as cancer and diabetes mellitus are major problems. Trends in the food supply of Egypt during the last twenty years are discussed. In spite of the apparent increased affluence of the population, there has been no improvement in the nutritional status in a decade. This may be due to increased food prices. Studies indicate that the educational level of mothers, independent of household income, is positively related to a better nutritional status of children. The authors conclude that general education and nutrition education are the main solutions.

In conclusion I would like to thank Professor Gabr for his advice, continuing encouragement, and editorial assistance. Despite his manifold national and international responsibilities, he devoted considerable time to the book.

MARGARET R. BISWAS
Chairman
Committee on Nutrition and Development
International Union of Nutritional Sciences
Oxford, England

# Contributors

SARAH J. ATKINSON
Urban Health Programme
London School of Hygiene and Tropical Medicine
Keppel Street
London WC1E 7HT
UK

MARGARET R. BISWAS
Biswas & Associates
76 Woodstock Close
Oxford OX2 8DD
UK.

MOHAMED EL-GHORAB
Nutrition Institute
Cairo
Egypt

MAMDOUH GABR
Department of Pediatrics
Cairo University
Egypt

C. GOPALAN
Nutrition Foundation of India
B-37 Gulmohar Park
New Delhi 110049
India

LAWRENCE HADDAD
International Food Policy Research Institute
1200 Seventeenth Street, N.W.
Washington, D.C. 20036
USA

BRIDGET H-H. HSU-HAGE
Department of Medicine
Monash Medical Centre
246 Clayton Road
Clayton
Vic 3168
Australia

MOHAMED AMR HUSSEIN
Nutrition Institute
Cairo
Egypt

EILEEN KENNEDY
International Food Policy Research Institute
1200 Seventeenth Street, N.W.
Washington, D.C. 20036
USA

WIDJAJA LUKITO
Department of Medicine
Monash Medical Centre
246 Clayton Road
Clayton
Vic 3168
Australia

WAFAA A. MOUSSA
Nutrition Institute
Cairo
Egypt

PAULINE PETERS
Harvard Institute for International Development
1 Elliot Street
Cambridge
Massachusetts 02138
USA

DAVID E. SAHN
Cornell University
Food and Nutrition Policy Program
Ithaca
New York 14853
USA

MARK L. WAHLQVIST
Department of Medicine
Monash Medical Centre
246 Clayton Road
Clayton
Vic 3168
Australia

# 1

# Nutrition, Food Production, and the Environment

MARGARET R. BISWAS

## INTRODUCTION

It is appropriate that the two conferences convened in 1992 by the United Nations at the ministerial level were on environment and development and on nutrition. The United Nations Conference on Environment and Development held in Rio in June was followed by the International Conference on Nutrition convened in Rome in December 1992. Eradicating hunger and malnutrition within the next decade, as recommended by the Nutrition Conference, is one of the most urgent environmental goals. In order to achieve this aim, the rapid growth of population in some developing countries must be addressed simultaneously. The increasing migration of rural inhabitants to urban areas, frequently slums, can make both the goals of nutrition and employment more difficult to achieve than in rural areas. Hence, the development of rural areas, with the purpose of discouraging migration to cities, is an equally important task.

The Green Revolution has enabled mankind to make remarkable strides in reducing hunger in the last three decades, especially in developing countries. There have also been negative side-effects which must be reduced, if not eliminated. Despite limited conservation efforts, the resources necessary for food production have shown a disquieting deterioration during the last two decades. Modern intensive agriculture has had an adverse effect not only on the physical environment but also on human health. Land has been degraded by salinity, waterlogging, and erosion. Water resources have been depleted while genetic resources have been lost. In addition, there have been negative impacts on human health because of agricultural inputs such as fertilizers, pesticides, and irrigation.

Agricultural inputs are just a few of the many chemical and biological contaminants of food and water. Most cases of ill-health and premature death continue to be caused by biological agents in the environment in food, water, and soil.

A majority of these environmental problems can be resolved, but the phenomenal growth of populations, especially in some developing countries, renders it very difficult to implement the solutions.

## POPULATION

Excessive population growth is one of the foremost contributory causes of environmental degradation. It compounds all the others, ranging from malnutrition and shortage of arable land, to toxicity in the air, water, and the foodchain. The more people there are, the more persons will there be in need of food at the global, national, and household levels. It will also become progressively more difficult to feed them for a variety of reasons, including limited availability of arable land, part of which is often required for construction of roads, houses, and other infrastructure. The poor are often confined to marginal land, perpetuating their poverty and degrading the land. The population problem needs urgent attention in countries where it is likely to double within the next two decades.

Controlling the spawning of population results in less need for more food. In fact, in many countries any gains in food production continue to be offset by population growth. A smaller population allows more financial resources for social and economic infrastructure such as employment, health, and education. Excessive population growth destroys the functioning of the existing social and physical infrastructure, including the ecosystem.

The United Nations Population Fund (UNFPA, 1992) predicts that world population will increase to 6 billion in 1998 from 5.48 billion in mid-1992 (Fig. 1.1). During the next decade, world population is estimated to grow by 97 million per year. Over half of this increase will occur in Africa and South Asia. This means that the absolute number of poor will multiply, and therefore also the number of malnourished. FAO estimates the number of malnourished will soar to 590 million by the year 2000 (WHO, 1992).

Poverty in rural areas is responsible for the migration of many individuals to urban areas or to other countries that offer the hope of better

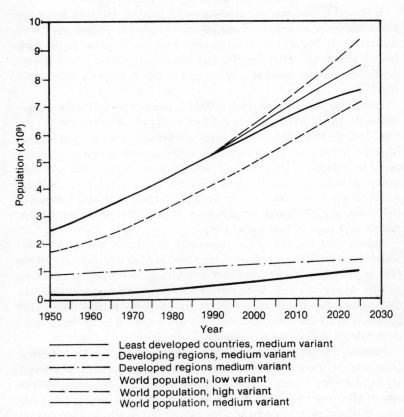

**Fig. 1.1** World population trends and projections, 1950–2025

Source: World population prospects 1990. United Nations, New York, 1991
(document ST//SA/SER A/120)

diet, health, and sanitation. An increasing number, however, are being crowded into urban slums and exposed to malnutrition and infectious diseases. Some 83 per cent of population growth in the next decade is expected to be in the urban milieu (UNFPA, 1992), partially due to migration from rural areas. This staggering increase in city-dwellers will pose acute problems in terms of nutrition, as discussed in the chapter on 'Food Security and Poor Urban Populations'. Malnutrition will continue to be the bane of vulnerable groups in low-income households, often in slums.

It is well known that the elimination of poverty will help to resolve the problems of malnutrition and population growth. People must have not only food, but also essential services such as education, health care, family planning, water supply, and sanitation. Employment opportunities for women must also be created as this helps to reduce family size.

According to the World Bank (1992), avoiding conception for women under the age of 20 could reduce the mortality of under-fives by 17 per cent. Spacing births at least two years apart could save the same number of lives. If these two measures were implemented, maternal mortality could be reduced by 40 per cent. This, however, implies access to contraception which frequently does not meet the demand. Neglected demand ranges from about 15 per cent of couples in Brazil, Colombia, Indonesia, and Sri Lanka to more than 35 per cent in Bolivia, Ghana, Kenya, and Togo (World Bank, 1992).

Survey data reveal that the percentage of married women who demand contraception range from 6.4 per cent in Mali to a high of 33.9 per cent in Kenya, 30–50 per cent in North Africa, 36–55 per cent in Asia, and 40–60 per cent in South America (Cleaver and Schreiber, 1992). In many cases, family planning officers do not perform their duties efficiently, if at all. Even in India, rarely is any action taken by the government against such erring individuals.

Female education is also of paramount importance. Data from a cross-section of countries indicate that where no women attend secondary school, they have an average of seven children, but where 40 per cent of all women have had a secondary education, the average drops to three children, even when the income factor is taken into account (World Bank, 1992). In Bangladesh, female enrolment in secondary education almost doubled as the result of one scholarship programme, with consequent lowering of fertility. The late President Ziaur Rahman of Bangladesh planned, before his untimely death in 1981, to install battery-operated television sets in every village to facilitate reading, and thereby to eradicate illiteracy in five years (Biswas and Biswas, 1981).

## Per Capita Food Supply

While positive strides have been made in lowering fertility, even more revolutionary advances have been made in food production, mainly through the development of high-yielding varieties. In the last two decades in China, India, and Indonesia, the three most populous countries of the developing world, annual growth rates of food production have exceeded those of population growth (World Bank, 1992). Meanwhile, in many other low-income countries, food production has barely kept pace with population growth. In Africa, per capita food production has declined by an average of 1 per cent a year during the last three decades (UNICEF, 1989).

As indicated in Table 1.1, the index of per capita agricultural production in Africa actually declined significantly from 108.90 in 1974 to 90.35 in 1990 (1979–81=100). During the same period in Asia, the index climbed from 92.06 to 118.84. If the two most populous countries of the world are considered, China fared much better than India: per capita index of agricultural production in China improved from 90.49 to 136.66, whereas in India the corresponding increase was from 91.00 to 119.07 (Table 1.1). In South America and Europe, the per capita index rose steadily during this period.

The global per capita food supply per day showed a steady upward trend during the 1969–88 period (Table 1.2). In terms of calories, per capita food supply per day increased from 2434 during 1969–71 to 2671 by 1986–88: a corresponding increase from 64.6 to 70.0. was registered in terms of protein/g. The general trend in different regions, including Africa, was one of steady increase, though the growth rates and the bases from which they increased differed from one region to another. For example, in terms of calories, the per capita average in Africa during 1969–71 was higher than that of Asia: 2121 calories as against 2087 calories. However, by 1986–88, Asia had overtaken Africa by 2450 ca-

**Table 1.1** Per capita agricultural production indices, with 1979–81=100

|             | 1974   | 1977   | 1982   | 1987   | 1990   |
|-------------|--------|--------|--------|--------|--------|
| World       | 96.56  | 98.31  | 102.21 | 102.94 | 104.37 |
| Africa      | 108.90 | 102.07 | 98.75  | 93.12  | 90.35  |
| N.C. America| 90.14  | 99.31  | 101.66 | 92.84  | 94.71  |
| S. America  | 95.41  | 99.49  | 101.55 | 101.19 | 102.48 |
| Asia        | 92.06  | 95.30  | 104.42 | 112.87 | 118.84 |
| China       | 90.49  | 87.34  | 110.17 | 131.19 | 136.66 |
| India       | 91.00  | 103.93 | 100.34 | 104.79 | 119.07 |
| Europe      | 94.52  | 93.58  | 103.96 | 106.88 | 105.01 |
| Oceania     | 93.65  | 100.21 | 92.42  | 97.85  | 97.33  |
| USSR        | 104.84 | 103.93 | 102.76 | 109.68 | 112.25 |

Source: Compiled from various FAO data sources

**Table 1.2** Per capita food supply per day

|  | 1969–71 | | 1974–76 | | 1982–84 | | 1986–88 | |
|---|---|---|---|---|---|---|---|---|
|  | Calories | Prot./g | Calories | Prot./g | Calories | Prot./g | Calories | Prot./g |
| World | 2434 | 64.6 | 2467 | 65.3 | 2642 | 68.6 | 2671 | 70.0 |
| Africa | 2121 | 53.0 | 2159 | 53.1 | 2238 | 54.3 | 2261 | 55.0 |
| N.C. America | 3109 | 91.6 | 3134 | 91.0 | 3285 | 93.1 | 3371 | 96.2 |
| Asia | 2087 | 51.5 | 2141 | 52.7 | 2421 | 58.8 | 2450 | 60.4 |
| Europe | 3250 | 93.4 | 3312 | 96.8 | 3372 | 100.1 | 3459 | 103.3 |
| Oceania | 3008 | 88.5 | 3037 | 89.0 | 3099 | 88.9 | 3149 | 90.3 |

Source: Compiled from various FAO sources

lories to 2261 calories. In terms of protein, the trend was similar to that observed with calories. The food supply includes food aid and imports.

According to UNICEF (1989), over the last decade the requisite expertise has been acquired to double the food production of small farms in Africa. New varieties of African maize, cowpeas, and cassava have been bred. Techniques of inter-cropping and nitrogen fixation, as well as conservation measures, have been developed. Proven technical advances need to be implemented, with emphasis on small farms and rural development, including family planning and health care.

It is probable that the increasing numbers of malnourished in Africa can be fed if the projected potential for irrigation can be realized. Studies on African development problems by multilateral and bilateral aid agencies have been undertaken for decades, but the data have frequently been taken home by the foreign researchers. Africans have been educated, and in many nations they are in a position to conduct adaptive research and implement the results. Extension services, however, remain a problem in all developing countries.

In many Asian countries, arable land and shortage of water will emerge as major constraints with regard to food production in the future while a lack of employment continues as the major reason for malnutrition.

## Population and Land Use

The relationship between population and availability of arable land is complex, since both features are dynamic and affected by many interrelated factors. For example, availability of arable land in any country, at any specific time, depends on technology, economics, land tenure pat-

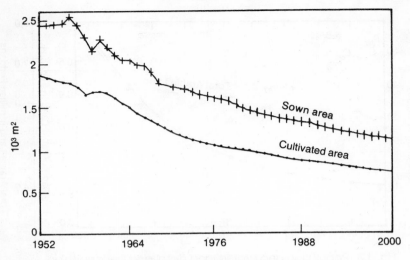

**Fig. 1.2** Per capita cultivated and sown area in China

terns, and environmental factors such as desertification and patterns of development. Thus, major water development projects, such as the Aswan High Dam in Egypt and the Indira Gandhi Canal Project in India, enabled these countries to increase the availability of arable land. Simultaneously, urban and rural growth and transportational infrastructure steadily reduced the availability of arable land.

As a general rule, in nearly all developing countries, arable land available per capita has steadily declined with time because of high population growth. Thus, in China, the most populous country in the world, there was 0.188 ha of cultivated land and 0.246 ha of sown area per person in 1952. By 1990, the corresponding figures had declined to 0.086 ha and 0.129 ha respectively (Economic Research Service, 1990). The changing pattern of per capita cultivated land and sown areas in China during the period 1952–2000 is shown in Fig. 1.2. By comparison, each person in the United States is supported by 0.735 ha of cropland, which is more than eight times that of China.

Between 1952 and 1990, cultivated land in China declined by nearly 12 per cent, whereas sown area increased by 2.1 per cent. Three basic forces—self preservation, state orders, and market forces—changed the agricultural land-use pattern in China. Land area used for planting grain

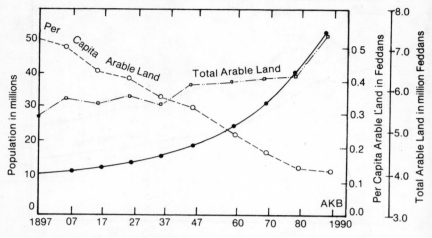

**Fig. 1.3** Population and arable land (total and per capita) in Egypt, 1897–1990 (Biswas, 1991)

crops declined from 124 million ha in 1952 to 111 million ha in 1990, an annual average decrease of 2.1 per cent. During the same period, areas under economic crops increased by 69 per cent, from 12.5 million ha to 21.1 million ha, and areas under other crops increased by 142 per cent, from 4.8 million ha to 11.5 million ha. Figure 1.3 shows similar changes in Egypt in terms of population, total arable land, and per capita arable land (Biswas, 1991).

## AGRICULTURE AND EMPLOYMENT

Agriculture does not only provide food but is also a source of income to farmers and landless labourers, enabling them to buy more food and other essentials. This makes it doubly imperative that we sustain the resources that support agriculture. Globally, in 1965, nearly 57.6 per cent of economically-active populations were engaged principally in agricultural activities (Table 1.3). By 1989, this percentage had declined to 47 per cent. Second, the rates of decline varied from region to region. The declines observed in Asia and Africa were somewhat similar: around 12.5 per cent. Third, the percentages of people engaged principally in agriculture in developing countries were much higher than in

**Table 1.3** Percentage of economically-active population engaged principally in agriculture, forestry, hunting or fishing

|            | 1965 | 1970 | 1975 | 1980 | 1985 | 1989 |
|------------|------|------|------|------|------|------|
| World      | 57.6 | 55.0 | 52.8 | 50.8 | 48.7 | 47.0 |
| Africa     | 76.4 | 74.4 | 71.5 | 68.7 | 66.0 | 63.7 |
| N.C. America | 15.8 | 14.0 | 13.1 | 12.2 | 11.4 | 10.9 |
| S. America | 41.2 | 38.1 | 33.4 | 28.8 | 25.9 | 23.7 |
| Asia       | 72.7 | 70.2 | 67.9 | 65.7 | 62.9 | 60.5 |
| Europe     | 24.0 | 19.9 | 16.8 | 13.7 | 11.0 | 9.7  |
| Oceania    | 24.6 | 22.5 | 20.9 | 19.6 | 18.0 | 16.8 |
| USSR       | 33.8 | 25.7 | 22.8 | 20.0 | 16.2 | 13.6 |

Source: Compiled from various FAO sources

developed countries. For example, in 1989, only 2.9 per cent of the U.S. population were engaged in agricultural activities as against 91.8 per cent in Nepal and 90.9 per cent in Bhutan. Regionally, in 1989, both Africa and Asia had the largest percentages of people engaged in agriculture, 63.7 per cent and 60.5 per cent, respectively. Even in an industrializing lower-middle-income country such as Thailand, agriculture continues to be the main source of livelihood (ACC/SCN, 1989).

In addition, processing, distribution, and marketing of food create an amazing number of jobs—even in developed countries. While urbanization undoubtedly lowers the percentage of employment in agriculture, the absolute number of employees definitely increases due to population growth. Hence, it is of utmost importance that the maximum potential of existing resources for food production be realized while sustaining their productivity for the future.

## The Role of Women

Women have worked in agriculture throughout history, but it is only in the last two decades that their role has been recognized. This has led, in recent years, to some studies on their role and work in most developing countries, including the implications for nutrition.

Recognition and research has so far had limited practical results at the farm level. The number of trained women has been increasing, as has their access to inputs in some areas. Development agencies have taken a lead, but much more attention to this field will be required in the coming decades.

In Africa, women continue to produce 70 per cent of the staple food and, in parts, form 60–90 per cent of the agricultural labour force. As men migrate to cities to work, women manage 50 per cent of the farms in many rural areas (World Resources Institute, 1990). Men, however, continue to possess the land titles, with the result that women have not had necessary access to credit for purchase of agricultural inputs. This has meant agricultural production, and hence family nutrition and income levels have not been as high as otherwise have been possible.

The introduction of irrigated agriculture has, in many countries, increased the workload of women due to many reasons (Biswas, 1987). First, the introduction of irrigation often means that two to three crops can be grown every year, instead of one. Weeding for irrigated farming is done mostly by women: generally very little or no weeding is necessary for dry farming. Second, as farm incomes increase, livestock holdings multiply as well. Since women are primarily responsible for the animals, extra work needs to be carried out every day. This may, however, increase the food supply, improving the nutritional status. The increased crop residues and dung will be used for cooking. This reduces the need for fuelwood, saving time and money for women as well as forest resources. On the other hand, if they are overburdened by farm work, women tend to keep children out of school to help and are reluctant to limit the size of their families. Ill-educated girls then marry young and perpetuate the poverty-stricken lifestyle.

## GREEN REVOLUTION

In view of the limited new land in the last two decades, increased production had to be gained from bigger yields through technical innovations. The Green Revolution may be credited with a major share of the rapid increase in food production since 1965. High-yielding varieties are responsible for the significant gains in rice and wheat production in Asia, Africa, Latin America, and the Mediterranean nations. Even in England, plant breeding accounted for about 65 per cent of the increase in wheat yields over the 25 years from 1960 to 1975. Half of the trebling of maize yields in the United States in the past 45 years is due to plant breeding (OECD, 1991). Africa can solve a major portion of its food deficit by introducing more high-yielding varieties, as discussed earlier.

The Green Revolution in wheat and rice has saved land through an improvement in yield per hectare. In 1964, India produced 12 million tonnes of wheat on 14 million ha. In 1990, after the introduction of high-yielding varieties, Indian farmers harvested about 55 million tonnes of wheat from about 23 million ha. In order to produce tonnes of wheat at 1964 (pre-Green Revolution) yield levels, India would have needed at least an additional 40 million ha of land (Swaminathan, 1991).

The Green Revolution has inadvertently had adverse impacts on both human nutrition and the environment. The extra income generated in rural areas has not always served to boost the nutritional status of rural populations. The diversion of land from grain legumes to cereals in India has caused a decline in protein consumption. Furthermore, small farmers often cannot afford the necessary inputs. They must be given access to these inputs, if food production is to be maximized, and thereby adequate food provided.

Mechanization and other technologies have often displaced the traditional jobs of women (Swaminathan, 1991a). This is true for the substitution of the application of organic manure with mineral fertilizers. Women have also been the traditional seed-selectors in poor countries. Heavy machinery can degrade fragile soil. The high-yielding varieties, which have in some cases supplanted native varieties now in danger of extinction, are often less resistant to pests and diseases. For example, the spread of high-yielding varieties of wheat and rice since the mid-1960s has caused a loss of the gene pools in centres of crop diversity such as Afghanistan, Iran, Iraq, Pakistan, and Turkey (El-Hinnawi, 1991). The extensive cultivation of a few crops has multiplied the number of pests and diseases by providing ideal conditions for their spread.

High-yielding varieties also require pesticides, fertilizers, and irrigation to reach their full potential. These inputs have both positive and negative impacts on the environment. (The effects are discussed in the following section.) Both fertilizers and pesticides have often been used excessively. A gradual termination of subsidies has helped to curb this abuse in some countries.

## PESTICIDES

Pesticide use has increased in many countries, but decreased in others such as the United States, Egypt, and Brazil during the decade 1975–84. Pesticides are increasingly applied to fruits and vegetables to assure high quality products in most countries.

The use of pesticides for cosmetic purposes is a negative development in terms of the environment and human health (Pimentel *et al.*, 1991). Their success in controlling pests on a short-term basis cannot be denied, but their long-term effectiveness in controlling pests and their overall effects on the ecosystems (including human health) could be seriously questioned. After the Second World War, the use of organochlorine pesticides was intensified. In contrast to the organophosphate group of pesticides that are biodegradable, organochlorines do not easily decompose. They are gradually dispersed to ecosystems other than the targeted one by drainage waters, or by evaporation and subsequent precipitation, becoming hazardous to humans in food, water and other ways.

In industrialized countries, some of these pesticides were banned in the late seventies and replaced by organophosphates and carbamates. Though some of these compounds are toxic, they do not accumulate in humans or the environment to any significant degree. Modern herbicides and fungicides are not very toxic and are not known to harm human health (Conway and Pretty, 1991). This is also true for synthetic pyrethroids.

Perhaps the most disturbing side-effect of the use of pesticides is.the unfortunate consequences for human beings. In the United States, the use of agricultural pesticides causes approximately 20,000 accidental poisonings every year, resulting in about 50 deaths (Pimentel *et al.*, 1991). In developing countries, illness and mortality due to pesticide poisoning is even more marked due to such factors as inappropriate handling and inaccurate labelling. Furthermore, pesticides banned in developed nations have, in the past, often been sold in developing countries; examples include endrin, parathion, and mevinphos (WHO, 1992).

The extent of carcinogenicity among pesticides remains a controversial issue (Conway and Pretty, 1991). The World Health Organization regards the risks of carcinogenicity as minimal. On the other hand, the United States Environmental Protection Agency has identified 53 compounds as causing either benign or malignant tumours. These are, however, mostly pesticides produced before 1970.

Pesticide residues in food products, on the other hand, remain an unresolved problem as the research required to determine their impact on health has not yet been conducted. The effects of low doses of pesticide use over long periods have not been ascertained. Pesticide residues can also accumulate in the soil, contaminating crops and ruining the fertility of the soil. Within ecosystems, there is an increasing concentration of pesticide residues as they move up the foodchain.

The intake of DDT by infants in Delhi is about 12 times more than the accepted daily intake of DDT (Zaidi *et al.*, 1989). This reflects the fact that pesticide residues are eliminated through mothers' milk. The

DDT and HCH levels are generally on the decline but remain high in humans and animals in Delhi.

Other side-effects include those on non-target organisms such as birds and fish. Pesticides may destroy parasites and predators of pests that were innocuous prior to the application of pesticides, resulting in outbreaks. The continued large-scale use of pesticides has resulted, through natural selection and evolution processes, in new strains of resistant species which generally turn out to be more vicious than their original counterparts. FAO states that resistant species of insects and mites have increased from 182 in 1965 to 288 in 1968 and to 428 in 1980 (OECD, 1991).

In 1985, the FAO Conference approved an International Code of Conduct on the Distribution and Use of Pesticides to regulate their use and marketing. Igbedioh (1991) states that developing nations should establish Pesticide Monitoring Agencies to control all aspects of sale, use, transport, and disposal of pesticides. Using unsuitable plastic containers for pesticides may result in spillage. Furthermore, they are often used by people for storing drinking water.

## Integrated Pest Management

The pesticide problems confronting the world need to be resolved through integrated pest management (IPM), combining the optimum methods of biological, chemical, mechanical, and other means of control. Other measures undertaken to integrate pest control might include releasing biological control agents, pest-specific diseases, or, when necessary, applying pesticides in limited amounts. Release of sterile males, or artificially-reared natural enemies of the pest, has proved successful in controlling a number of insect pests. Other methods of intervention include choice of sowing, weeding, and harvesting time, location of fields, crops rotation, destruction of crop remains, selection of more resistant crop varieties, and breeding new varieties of plants that are resistant to pests and diseases.

Total agricultural pesticide use in the United States for 42 major crops could be reduced by 50 per cent by applying integrated pest management (Pimentel et al., 1991). Scandinavian countries and the Netherlands have already undertaken a 50 per cent reduction of their pesticide use.

Programmes introducing IPM are being developed in various Asian countries with varying degrees of success. IPM, which is more complex than chemical control, requires training. Rice farmers in the Philippines and Indonesia have, however, rapidly acquired the IPM expertise during government-sponsored programmes (Kenmore *et al.*, 1987). Lack of financing and institutional support are major constraints in the implementation of IPM in developing countries. Given the ineffectiveness of most extension services in these regions, the feasibility of IPM is likely to be limited in the near future.

## FERTILIZERS

The use of fertilizers and pesticides is one of the major factors contributing to the doubling of the world's cereal production during the last 30 years. Far more accurate data are available for fertilizers than for pesticides. In 1989, Asia accounted for 31 per cent of the total annual global fertilizer consumption and nearly 40 per cent of nitrogen use. In contrast, Africa's share of both the total annual global fertilizer and nitrogen consumption was less than 3 per cent in 1989. Per hectare fertilizer use in Africa in 1989 at 3.8 kg was only about one per cent the usage rate of Japan (365.4 kg) and less than 3 per cent of that of the United States (143.9 kg). In Latin America, the usage rate was 9.4 kg by 1989, which even though more than double the 1973 rate, was still low. In contrast, fertilizer use in Asia nearly quadrupled from 14.1 kg per ha in 1973 to 66.7 kg per ha in 1989.

It should also be noted that in the developing countries most of the fertilizers and pesticides are applied to irrigated areas, even though agriculture is largely practised in rain-fed land. Thus, the potential for increasing agricultural production in rain-fed areas of the developing countries through higher use of fertilizers is indeed very significant.

Increased use of fertilizers is an especially important consideration for most developing countries where regular fertilizer losses are incurred due to annual cropping and leaching. FAO (1990) studies indicate that a country like Zimbabwe alone could be losing 1.6 million tonnes of nitrogen, 0.24 million tonnes of phosphorus, and 15.6 million tonnes of organic matter every year due to soil erosion. Clearly, nutrients lost to the soil have to be replaced regularly and adequately to ensure its productivity.

### Environmental Effects

Fertilizers are indispensable for increasing food production, but their excessive and inefficient use has occasioned much concern as a possible environmental threat. Chief among these concerns are the contributions of phosphate and nitrogen fertilizers to eutrophication, and higher concentration of nitrogen in water. A primary environmental concern in recent years has been the high level of nitrogen concentration in drinking water, which is especially dangerous for infants under the age of six months.

Methaemoglobinaemia in infants has been traced to high nitrate intakes in parts of the industrialized countries, but has rarely been diagnosed in the tropics, where conditions are even more conducive to its persistence: infants drink more liquids because of the heat, diarrhoea is common, and diets are poor in vitamin C (WHO, 1978). Undoubtedly, methaemoglobinaemia prevails, but health personnel are either unaware of its symptoms or infants die from diarrhoea before methaemoglobinaemia reaches the advanced stages. In the United States, bottled water is made available for babies where local drinking water has high nitrate levels. For instance, in 38 towns in Nebraska, where domestic water supply shows high nitrate concentrations, babies are given bottled water (Biswas, 1990). In the developing countries, however, widespread poverty does not make this a feasible solution.

Nitrates are also believed to cause cancer, especially gastric cancer. While there is some evidence of a relationship between gastric cancer and nitrates in food and drinking water, the link has not been established. There may also be an association with bladder cancer, common in Egypt, and oesophageal cancer prevalent in northern China (Conway and Pretty, 1991).

An overdose of fertilizer in food crops sometimes causes large concentrations of nitrates to leach into groundwater. Once groundwater is contaminated, it cannot be easily or economically purified. Generally, if fertilizer is used efficiently at recommended levels, little leaching occurs. The problem of nitrate pollution of water from agricultural sources has adversely affected human health in France, the Netherlands, the Federal Republic of Germany, and the United Kingdom (OECD, 1991).

To prevent excessive application of mineral fertilizers, organic fertilizers should be used in an integrated programme. Crop residues, manure, and biological nitrogen fixation can be combined with a supplement of mineral fertilizer.

## IRRIGATION DEVELOPMENT AND HEALTH

Irrigated agricultural projects, which are expected to increase food supply and thereby improve the nutritional status of the recipients, often have an adverse impact on human health instead of improving it as planned. Such thwarted aims have placed the focus during the past two decades on vector-borne diseases, especially schistosomiasis and malaria (WHO, 1990). There is no doubt that the presence of an irrigation system in warm climates, with extended shorelines of reservoirs and canal banks, contributes to a more optimal habitat for the vectors of schistosomiasis and malaria. While this is a scientific fact, it has not yet been determined to what extent the irrigated practices *per se* contribute to the incidence of schistosomiasis and malaria.

On the basis of the few available studies, only limited conclusions may be drawn. Research in Egypt and South and South-East Asia has revealed that much of the schistosomiasis infection occurs not during the irrigation phase, but during other contacts with impure water, especially when domestic water supply and sanitation are sub-standard. The provision of clean water, sanitation, better health care, and health education is significantly reducing the incidence of schistosomiasis. A good example is Egypt, which has been afflicted with schistosomiasis since Pharaonic times. With the implementation of the aforementioned safeguards, it is expected that, by the year 2000, schistosomiasis will no longer be endemic (Biswas, 1992).

Similarly, detailed district-by-district study in India indicates that there is no direct correlation between the annual parasitic index of malaria and the presence or absence of irrigation (Sharma, 1987). Sharma and his colleagues have developed an interesting approach to containing malaria (Malaria Research Centre). The document *Malaria and Development in Africa*, produced by the American Association for the Advancement of Science, provides a discussion of the approach required to deal with the complexities of malaria. While it is true that irrigation projects may be linked with malaria, there are evidently factors other than irrigation that are more responsible for malarial incidence. Poor drainage contributes to the spread of all types of vector-borne diseases in irrigation development. Rigorous scientific studies are urgently needed for better understanding of the complex interrelationships between agriculture, environment, and health.

## LAND DEGRADATION

Irrigation not only increases the productivity of land, it also contributes to land degradation due to the development of salinity and waterlogging.

While waterlogging is not an inevitable result of irrigation, it occurs because of inadequate provision of drainage. Soil salinity increases since plants extract pure water and most of the salt contained in irrigated water is left behind. It should be noted that the techniques for preventing the development of waterlogging and salinity are well known, but for a variety of reasons they have not been applied.

Soil scientists have established that the world is now losing about 1.5 million ha of irrigated lands *annually* mainly due to salinization in the drylands (UNEP, 1992). It is further estimated that erosion and urbanization are largely responsible for the annual loss of about 7–8 million ha of rainfed croplands in the world. Over half of this degradation has occurred in the drylands.

UNEP defines land degradation in arid, semi-arid, and dry subhumid areas (drylands), resulting mainly from adverse human impact, as desertification. Land, in this context, includes soil and local water resources, land surface, vegetation, and crops (UNEP, 1992). During the last two decades, recurrent drought, and inappropriate management of natural resources, especially in Africa, have threatened the lives of millions of dryland inhabitants. In developing countries, these drylands (unlike those in industrialized countries) are the basis of agricultural production. Desertification has been a prime cause of the migration of subsistence farmers and pastoralists to urban areas where they often have to contend with even more questionable nutrition.

The 1990 UNEP assessment indicates that the situation continues to deteriorate (see Table 1.4). At present, nearly 3.6 billion ha (or about 70 per cent) of drylands are exposed to degradation of natural vegetation, and also soil deterioration. The most extensive areas of degraded drylands are in Asia.

Not only in drylands but on other land also, demands for production have increased the pressure on existing land and the utilization of mar-

**Table 1.4** Land degradation

|  | Desertification (million ha) | |
| --- | --- | --- |
|  | 1984 | 1990 |
| 1. Degraded irrigated lands | 40 | 43 |
| 2. Degraded rainfed croplands | 335 | 216 |
| 3. Degraded rangelands | 3100 | 3333 |
| 4. Total degraded drylands | 3475 | 3592 |

Source: UNEP, 1992

ginal lands. Extensive areas of traditional pasture land have been cultivated, with herders moving on. These factors have sometimes resulted in
rapid land degradation with subsequent decline in production, which, in
turn, reduce the nutritional status of already vulnerable populations. Cultivation of steep hillsides and shifting cultivation have led to deforesta-
tion, soil erosion, sedimentation, and floods, destroying the basis for
production.

Counter-measures to land degradation are well-known. Contour cultivation, reforestation, mulching, appropriate land tenure, and alternative
employment to agriculture are among the many essential measures implemented to preserve land where it is most needed.

## MICRONUTRIENT DEFICIENCIES AND THE ENVIRONMENT

Plants grow by absorbing water and nutrients from the soil. Depleted
soils can therefore result in micronutrient deficiency in food. Furthermore, the mineral requirements of growing plants differ both quantita-
tively and qualitatively from those of humans and animals, subjecting
the latter to various nutrition problems. There is often a lack of sufficient
trace elements in the soil for their needs. For example, plants do not
require iodine and selenium, and may grow normally while lacking sufficient levels of these elements which are necessary for humans and
animals who consume the plants (Allaway, 1986).

Different species of some plants absorb different levels of trace elements (Allaway, 1986). Different strains of ryegrass accumulate varying
concentrations of iodine from the same soil. Different species of corn
accumulate varied levels of zinc when growing in the same soil. The
same is true for soybeans and selenium. Currently, no new varieties of
crops have been developed for the sole purpose of increasing human or
animal intake of essential trace elements. Wheat from central Canada
and the United States may have made a major contribution to preventing
selenium deficiency in populations of wheat-importing countries.

The realization that iodine deficiencies in soil and water cause the
health disorder goitre has resulted in supplementation in the form of
iodized salt to eliminate the deficiency in affected populations of many
nations. The discovery of the relationship between selenium levels in
local foods and Keshan disease in China has eliminated that affliction. These are the two confirmed relationships between trace element levels
in soils, plants, and health.

Recent research has been examining interrelationships of trace elements. It provides evidence that selenium deficiency impairs the utilization of iodine by humans. Selenium is a component of the enzyme that converts thyroxine to triiodothyroxine (Arthur, Nicol, and Beckett, 1990).

In Bangladesh, some food items, including milk, are deficient in some essential trace elements such as copper and zinc (Khan *et al.*, 1989). Zinc deficiency (Mannan and Rahim, 1988) in fruits, vegetables, legumes, grains, grasses, and fodder crops in Bangladesh is a major problem but the deficiency is more pronounced in rice crops grown on alkaline, wet, and waterlogged soils.

In India, the same problem is very much in evidence: 53% of both soils and crops in Andhra Pradesh, 50% in Punjab, and 64% in Haryana are deficient in zinc (Kanwar, 1990). These soils are also deficient in iron and manganese, but of a lower order. Zinc deficiency in soils and plants has emerged, in the wake of intensive application of modern agricultural technology, as a factor of major consequence.

According to Gopalan (1991), zinc deficiency could have a possible bearing on three of the major nutritional deficiency problems of South East Asia, namely, protein–energy malnutrition, hypovitaminosis A, and anaemia. Deficiency in zinc, a component of many key enzymes involved in protein synthesis, could aggravate PEM and contribute to growth retardation. It may be a factor in the pathogenesis of hypovitaminosis A. The greater vulnerability of the rice crop to zinc deficiency could be reflected in the poorer zinc nutritional status of rice consumers of Bangladesh and the eastern part of India. This could partly explain the more pronounced endemicity of vitamin A deficiency in these regions rather than in the wheat-consuming areas of western and northern India.

The use of refined fertilizers alone, without the addition of manure and cultivation of leguminous crops to replace certain nutrients, can alter, over time, the presence of micronutrients in the soil. This could result in loss of selenium, iron, copper, zinc, and manganese, with a consequent decline in crop yields as well as wide-ranging effects in human nutrition, which are not yet fully understood (Gopalan, 1991). Fertilizers used earlier were less refined than those generally used now.

Unrefined fertilizers contain various trace elements as impurities. For example, phosphorus fertilizers contain iron, cadmium, selenium, and fluoride (Allaway, 1986). Various fertilizers have been used to correct deficiencies as, for example, copper fertilizer for copper deficiency.

Sometimes it is the individual's diet rather than the soil that is deficient in micronutrients. This is because different foods provide different micronutrients, whereas one single food may contain several micronutrients. A good example involves the three main micronutrient deficiencies of public health significance: iodine, iron, and vitamin A. Green, leafy vegetables and animal foods have an abundant supply of iron and vitamin A, while fish products contain vitamin A and iodine (ICN). These foods, rich in vitamins and minerals, should be added to diets in which 80 per cent of the calories are comprised of cereals.

A great deal of research is required to determine nutrient relationships in soil, plants, and humans, and possible intervention programmes need to be formulated to correct nutritional disorders in human populations.

## POST-HARVEST LOSSES

Reliable estimates of post-harvest losses are not available at present. Many of the current estimates of post-harvest losses are of the order of 20 per cent or more. Greeley (1987) points out that the estimate of total maximum loss of 37 per cent (while in no way substantiated) has been 'highly influential in promoting increased funding for post-harvest research and development'.

Loss of food can, however, be substantial, especially in developing countries, and few countries would face food shortage, except in time of drought or civil war, if post-harvest losses could be reduced. Insects, moisture, moulds, and rodents can destroy rice, other cereals, cash crops such as sugar, and fruits and vegetables in storage. In the tropics and semi-tropics, mycotoxins, especially aflatoxins, attack cereals, groundnuts, some fruits, and tree nuts in storage. This deprives countries of exports and incurs financial losses which could be used for development.

In Asia, rodents spread such maladies as leptospirosis, Aujeszky's disease, diarrhoea, salmonellosis, and enteric fever by contaminating goods with urine and droppings (Mill, 1992). Food contamination in general is discussed in the next section.

The deprivation of the poor includes the lack of the means to defend their produce. Fortunately, simple technologies for improved storage, handling, and drying are being developed for use in developing countries. Proper handling through the stages of harvesting to marketing and consumption is essential. Small-scale processing in villages prevents losses by providing processed foods for transfer to urban areas. These measures will particularly benefit women who bear the main responsibility for storage and processing in rural areas.

## CONTAMINATION OF FOOD AND WATER

Any factor in the environment that reduces the intake of nutrients has a negative effect on the nutritional status, and thereby on the health of the individual. Furthermore, a seriously ill person cannot engage in productive employment.

Notwithstanding all the chemical pollution in modern times, most ill health and premature death continues to be caused by biological agents in the environment, in water, food, air, and soil (WHO, 1992). As discussed in the following sections, millions of people, mostly children in developing countries, die prematurely or fall ill due to pollution.

It should be noted that exposure to chemicals and radioactive material is a serious problem in both developed and developing countries. Intensive care is required if industrial pollution, including hazardous wastes, air pollution, heavy metals, and agricultural chemicals in food and water, is not to pose a risk to human health.

The number of diverse and innumerable pollutants in the environment has been increasing steadily in recent decades. The effects of most are not yet known, and the impacts of only a limited number have been ascertained. This chapter considers only those pollutants that contaminate food and water, for example, cadmium, lead, mercury, and arsenic. Pesticide residues, and how to limit their toxicity, have already been discussed in the section on pesticides.

## Chemical Pollutants

The discharge of large quantities of toxic metals into the air, water, and soils inevitably results in the transfer of pollutant metals to the human foodchain. This is even more true in developing countries where technology is old, often not properly maintained, and environmental control practices are not stringent. Even if there are fewer wastes in developing countries, disposal practices are often inadequate or non-existent. International assistance is required here and to deal with toxicity generally.

In developing countries, most food contamination is introduced during the local processing and marketing of the food products (Nriagu, 1992). Chemicals used in food processing and packing are also a matter of concern in industrialized nations.

In Africa, even some of the imported foods are not free of toxic metals. Imported food products, especially those from Asian and Latin

**Table 1.5** Concentrations (μg/g) of trace metals in human milk

| Element | Nigeria | Zaire | Guatemala | Hungary | Philippines | Sweden |
|---------|---------|-------|-----------|---------|-------------|--------|
| As | 1.8 | 0.26 | 0.29 | 0.24 | 19 | 0.55 |
| Cd | 3.7 | | | | 2.7 | |
| Co | 0.64 | 0.36 | 0.24 | 0.15 | 1.4 | 0.27 |
| Cr | 4.4 | 1.1 | 1.2 | 0.78 | 3.5 | 1.5 |
| Cu | 278 | 201 | 263 | 203 | 310 | 186 |
| Hg | 2.2 | 2.7 | 1.6 | 1.4 | 1.7 | 3.3 |
| Mo | 2.6 | 1.4 | 2.1 | | 16 | 0.4 |
| Ni | 12 | 4.9 | 12 | 14 | 16 | 11 |
| Pb | 4.9 | 5 | 2.9 | 15 | 17 | 17 |
| Sb | 4.1 | 3.6 | 1 | 1.6 | 11 | 3 |
| V | 0.46 | 0.27 | 0.21 | 0.11 | 0.69 | 0.13 |
| Zn | 1680 | 1920 | 2610 | 1200 | 1980 | 700 |

Source: Parr *et al.*, 1991

American countries, which may be sub-standard, arrive in metallic rather than glass or plastic containers.

Table 1.5 estimates the concentrations of trace metals in human milk. Lead levels are almost three times as high in Europe and the Philippines as in Zaire and Nigeria.

Improperly canned foods can contribute to the daily dietary intake of lead, but the main source of lead for urban populations is combustion of leaded petroleum from automobile exhausts. There is also lead emission into the atmosphere from manufacturing industries. Areas close to lead emissions have been found to have high lead concentration in forage crops and on the leaves of food crops (Allaway, 1986). Lead-carrying particles also contaminate soil and are absorbed by the roots of plants. Significant amounts may be consumed through water, when the piping for the supply is lead.

The effects of even low levels of lead (e.g. when a child picks it up in dust) on the central nervous system are of special concern (UNEP, 1992a). Many children in the urban areas of Africa are exposed to high daily doses of lead, often present in household dust, as compared with children in the temperate countries. Nriagu (1992) estimates that 19–30 per cent of the children in African cities suffer from lead poisoning. In adults, the blood, the gastrointestinal tract, and the nervous system are affected by high levels of lead.

Many countries have switched from lead-soldered to unsoldered cans so as to reduce the amount of lead in food. In Mexico, Kuwait, and African countries, lead poisoning from the use of inadequately glazed pots, pans, and cups is believed to be common (Nriagu, 1992). In western countries, the use of leaded gasoline is strictly limited. Of the developing countries, only a few, such as Thailand, Malaysia, and Mexico, are following this example.

Cadmium is also constantly being taken up by food crops after being deposited in the soil from the atmosphere. Cadmium is normally present in soils and contained in phosphate fertilizers in Europe and northern Africa. Cadmium in European topsoil has been increasing in recent decades.

Food contamination may also be caused by cadmium-plated and galvanized equipment in food processing (UNEP, 1992a). Industries, especially electroplating and battery manufacturing, release cadmium into the environment. In developing countries, small-scale electroplating and battery manufacturing industries do not have any special waste-treatment facilities. Industrial effluents are discharged into the domestic sewer systems, which are often incapable of properly treating significantly higher than designed effluent load. Accordingly, effluents discharged from sewerage treatment plants contain concentrated amounts of industrial chemicals and metals. This contributes to soil and water pollution. Such continual discharges build up the levels of environmental contamination and, at a certain stage, start to harm human health significantly.

Cadmium may cause increase in the incidence of prostatic and respiratory cancer. There is mounting evidence that it causes renal damage by accumulating in the kidneys (UNEP, 1992a).

One of the metals existing most widely in the environment is arsenic. Arsenic compounds have been used as pesticides for over a century; hence its toxicology is reasonably well understood (UNEP, 1992a). Contamination of food crops is low, but fish and shellfish may contain higher concentrations of organic arsenic, which are, however, of low toxicity. Inorganic arsenic is carcinogenic, especially to labourers in industry.

Mercury is discharged into water from industrial processes or may occur naturally. In water, it is transformed by micro-organisms into methylmercury, which is neurotoxic, and which, even at low levels of concentration, can harm the foetal brain. High concentrations are found in workers in the fishing industry and subsistence fishermen and populations whose diets include contaminated fish (WHO, 1992). Few reliable data are available on levels of mercury concentration or health effects in humans (UNEP, 1986).

UNEP (1992a) recommends that polychlorinated biphenyls (PCBs), which are used in a variety of industrial applications, be banned, except for essential uses, and replaced by substitutes. Despite the fact that their use has been restricted in many countries since the seventies (UNEP/FAO/WHO, 1988), their presence is still detected in the Arctic and Antarctic (UNEP, 1992a), where populations are exposed to the danger of infection. High levels of PCB have been found in fish from inland waters and enclosed seas, and in some countries in dairy products. Industrial workers face increased risk of cancer of the liver and biliary tract (Tomatis, 1990).

The same policy is recommended for curtailing the dispersion of heavy metals such as lead, mercury, and cadmium. New uses should be limited and recycling of metals encouraged. The developed countries must assist the developing countries in dealing with hazardous substances.

## Biological Contaminants

Varied biological contaminants, such as bacteria, viruses, moulds, and parasites, can cause a wide range of foodborne diseases from brucellosis to cholera and typhoid. Most diseases transmitted by contaminated food and water can cause diarrhoea. It has been estimated that contaminated food transmits as much as 70 per cent of all diarrhoea (Esrey and Feachem, 1989).

The practice of food-safety measures, such as pasteurization and proper processing, sanitation, clean water, and personal hygiene contribute to eliminating these biological factors. They remain problematical even in developed countries, causing hundreds of millions of cases of illness, many of which are fatal.

Figure 1.4 illustrates the rapid rise of infectious enteritis and the rapid decrease in typhoid and paratyphoid fevers in the decades since the Second World War in the Federal Republic of Germany.

There are several reasons for the existence of this significant contamination of food. The intensive livestock production, especially the rearing of pigs and poultry, has resulted in millions of animals becoming infected carriers of salmonella (WHO, 1992). They infect their environment—soils, water, etc.—and this environment has become the main source of infection of healthy animals. In some countries, 60–100% of poultry are infected with a variety of salmonella. Other foods are also contaminated by new strains of pathogens.

Another reason for infections is the increasing consumption of ready-

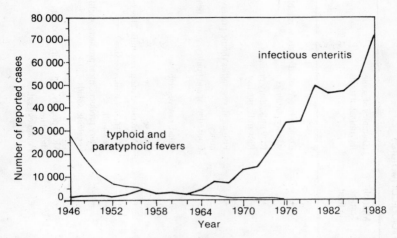

**Fig. 1.4** Infectious enteritis and typhoid and paratyphoid fevers in the Federal Republic of Germany, 1946–89 (WHO, 1992)

to-eat foods which are not handled with the necessary safety precautions. For instance, they must be stored at low temperatures and for short periods.

Table 1.6 provides some agents of foodborne diseases. Man emerges as the major carrier, with fish, dairy products, and meat as the foods most commonly contaminated.

Of particular concern in countries with hot, humid climates are mycotoxins which may not only result in intoxication, but have carcinogenic, mutagenic, and other effects on humans and animals. Of the hundreds of varieties, aflatoxin is the most dangerous from the point of view of public health. Epidemiological studies show a strong correlation between the high incidence of liver cancer and aflatoxin contamination of food.

## Food Safety Systems

In industrialized countries, food control systems ensure wholesome food, but in developing countries quality standards often remain low. Lack of legislation, and even more its implementation and monitoring, are major hurdles. Many nations lack trained personnel and laboratories

**Table 1.6** Some agents of foodborne disease and salient epidemiological features

| Agent | Important reservoir/carrier | Transmission[a] by | | | Multiplication in food | Examples of some incriminated foods |
|---|---|---|---|---|---|---|
| | | water | food | person-to-person | | |
| **BACTERIA** | | | | | | |
| *Bacillus cereus* | Soil | - | + | - | + | Cooked rice, cooked meats, vegetables, starchy puddings |
| *Brucella* spp | Cattle, goats, sheep | - | + | - | + | Raw milk, dairy products |
| *Campylobacter jejuni* | Chickens, dogs, cats, cattle, pigs, wild birds | + | + | + | -[b] | Raw milk, poultry |
| *Clostridium botulinum* | Soil, mammals, birds, fish | - | + | - | + | Fish meal, vegetables (home-preserved), honey |
| *Clostridium perfringens* | Soil, animals, man | - | + | - | + | Cooked meat and poultry, gravy, beans |
| *Escherichia coli* | | | | | | |
| Enterotoxigenic | Man | + | + | + | + | Salad, raw vegetables |
| Enteropathogenic | Man | + | + | + | + | Milk |
| Enteroinvasive | Man | + | + | O | + | Cheese |
| Enterohaemorrhagic | Cattle, poultry, sheep | + | + | + | + | Undercooked meat, raw milk, cheese |
| *Listeria monocytogenes* | Environment | + | + | -[c] | + | Cheese, raw milk, coleslaw |
| *Mycobacterium bovis* | Cattle | - | + | - | - | Raw milk |
| *Salmonella typhi* and *paratyphi* | Man | + | + | ± | + | Dairy products, meat products, shellfish, vegetable, salads |
| *Salmonella* (non-typhi) | Man and animals | ± | + | ± | + | Meat, poultry, eggs, dairy products, chocolate |
| *Shigella* spp | Man | + | + | + | + | Potato/egg salads |

| Organism | Reservoir | | | | | Foods/vehicles |
|---|---|---|---|---|---|---|
| Staphylococcus aureus (enterotoxins) | Man | − | + | − | + | Ham, poultry and egg salads, cream-filled bakery produce, ice-cream, cheese |
| Vibrio cholerae 01 | Man, marine life | + | + | ± | + | Salad, shellfish |
| Vibrio cholerae non-01 | Man, marine life | + | + | ± | + | Shellfish |
| Vibrio parahaemolyticus | Seawater, marine life | − | + | + | + | Raw fish, crabs, and other shellfish |
| Yersinia enterocolitica | Water, wild animals, pigs, | + | + | − | + | Milk, pork and poultry, dogs |
| **VIRUSES** | | | | | | |
| Hepatitis A virus | Man | + | + | + | − | Shellfish, raw fruit and vegetables |
| Norwalk agents | Man | + | + | + | − | Shellfish, salad |
| Rotavirus | Man | + | + | + | − | O |
| **PROTOZOA** | | | | | | |
| Cryptosporidium parvum | Man, animals | + | + | + | − | Raw milk, (non-fermented) sausage |
| Entamoeba histolytica | Man | + | + | + | − | Vegetables and fruits |
| Giardia lamblia | Man, animals | + | ± | ± | − | Vegetables and fruits |
| Toxoplasma gondii | Cats, pigs | O | + | + | − | Undercooked meat, raw vegetables |
| **HELMINTHS** | | | | | | |
| Ascaris lumbricoides | Man | + | + | + | − | Soil-contaminated food |
| Taenia saginata and T. solium | Cattle, swine | − | + | + | − | Undercooked meat |
| Trichinella spiralis | Swine, carnivora | − | + | + | − | Undercooked meat |
| Trichuris trichiura | Man | O | + | + | − | Soil-contaminated food |

+ = Yes; ± = Rare; − = No; O = No information

a Almost all acute enteric infections show increased transmission during the summer and/or wet months, except infections due to rotavirus and *Yersinia enterocolitica* which show increased transmission in cooler months.

b Under certain circumstances some multiplication has been observed. The epidemiological significance of this observation is not clear.

c Transmission from pregnant woman to foetus occurs frequently.

Source: Adapted from WHO Technical Report Series, No. 705, 1984 (The role of food safety in health and development: Report of a Joint FAO/WHO Expert Committee on Food Safety).

for chemicals and microbiological testing of foods. Since food contamination occurs all along the line from production to consumption, public awareness created by the media is also essential.

Unfortunately, food quality continues to have low priority in most developing nations (Igbedioh and Akinyele, 1992). The export of high quality foods in international markets will provide countries with the resources necessary for development. The standards of the FAO/WHO Codex Alimentarius Commission facilitate trade in food, protecting the consumer's health and ensuring fair trade practices. Sometimes, countries do not have the finances to introduce food safety systems. According to Igbedioh and Akinyele (1992), the overriding factor that determines whether a country will have effective food control is not so much financial constraints as the political will of the ruling government. They cite an uncompleted food training institute at Kaduna, Nigeria, and an unfinished laboratory at Maiduguri, Nigeria, as typical examples.

## WATER AND NUTRITION

Most of the human body is composed of water and good quality fresh water is essential for its functioning. Agriculture, industry, domestic work, and other activities require water. According to WHO (1992), nearly half the world's population suffers from diseases associated with insufficient or impure water. Ill-health caused by contaminated food or water afflicts mostly the poor in developing countries. Two billion people are at risk from diarrhoeal diseases caused by contaminated food and water, which are the principal cause of the death of nearly four million children annually.

The World Bank (1992) estimates that diarrhoeal disorders caused by contaminated water result in 900 million cases of illness each year and the death of two million children. In sub-Saharan Africa, contaminated drinking water and poor sanitation contribute to over 62 per cent of all deaths. This is twice the number in Latin America and twelve times that of industrialized countries. Drinking and washing in untreated water exposes people to disease from human wastes. Even in Morocco, the Minister of Health (1991) stated that over 85 per cent of all illnesses in Morocco were due to unclean water. This is a contributing factor to the malnutrition problem in Morocco.

Most of the diseases associated with food or water originate from human and animal wastes. Without treatment, they are transmitted to food and water. Cholera and typhoid are the most common waterborne diseases. Then there are diseases such as schistosomiasis and liver and lung flukes where water provides the habitat for the vector. Mosquitoes breed in water and are the vectors for malaria, filariasis, and viral infections such as dengue, yellow fever, and Japanese encephalitis. This proves that the battle against infectious diseases, malnutrition, and premature death will not be won without clean water. Unfortunately, access to potable water has barely kept pace with population growth. WHO figures estimate that during the International Drinking Water Supply and Sanitation Decade, 1980–90, over 1.6 billion additional people were provided with clean water (World Bank, 1992). Approximately 170 million city dwellers and over 855 million rural inhabitants (about a billion in total) continue to lack good quality water.

The number of people without sanitation increased throughout the Decade: 1.7 billion people had no access to sanitation globally, and the absolute number of people lacking such facilities increased by 70 million in urban areas. According to WHO (1990), 331 million urban dwellers and 1388 million rural inhabitants lack adequate sanitation. The least progress was observed in sub-Saharan Africa, where, due to high population growth, the percentage of urban people without access to clean water increased by about 29 per cent, in spite of the fact that the actual number of people receiving such services doubled. Similarly, the percentage of people in urban areas without sanitation facilities increased by 31 per cent, even though the number of people having such facilities had more than doubled.

Although additional sanitation has been provided, failure to treat human sewage has resulted in the deterioration of water quality. Poor maintenance of septic tanks can pollute groundwater, while piped sewerage systems can transmit infections to surface waters. The poor rely on surface water, lacking even the fuel to boil the water for drinking. Most urban areas in Africa and Asia have no sewerage systems, their untreated wastes landing in ditches, rivers, etc. (Hardoy and Satterthwaite, 1989). In Latin America, only two per cent of sewage receives any treatment (World Bank, 1992).

With the construction of more sewage treatment works in the cities of developing countries, large quantities of treated wastewater can be made available. This wastewater is an additional source of water. It can be used in agriculture, inland fisheries, industry, and groundwater recharge. These options increase with the extent of treatment and reliable quality control. And by reusing wastewater for appropriate purposes, higher quality water can be released for other purposes such as drinking.

The availability of usable wastewater in arid countries can be crucial. For example, Jordan has an extensive sewage-treatment plant construction programme which is expected to supply approximately 15 per cent of its total current water demand (Biswas and Arar, 1988).

## CONCLUSIONS

The progress in food production and the reduction of malnutrition in the last three decades have not occurred without some deterioration in the environment. While there has been a growing awareness of the need to sustain the resource base for agricultural production, implementation has been very limited. Known measures have not been taken by governments, farmers, and distributors. If the knowledge already available is put into practice, much will be achieved in terms of sustainable agriculture. In coming decades, preserving the environment will not be a choice, but an imperative, even in order to sustain the present rates of food production. Much greater efforts on behalf of the environment will have to be undertaken if the global population in the year 2000 is to have an adequate food supply.

If hunger and malnutrition are to be eradicated, the problem of population density will have to be addressed more seriously. Population growth in the next decade will be concentrated in Africa and South Asia. South Asia lacks land, and Africa has many other problems. Bad government, civil strife escalating to war, corruption, indebtedness, and the recession have added to agricultural problems such as drought, soil degradation, and lack of modern farming methods. The potential for increasing food production, however, exists. New crop varieties have been developed, and there is a pool of educated African professionals to assist in increasing production.

Another major environmental problem is the contamination of food and water by chemicals and biological agents. Food quality control laboratories, clean water, sanitation, and sewage treatment are essential to solve these critical problems in developing countries. Even in industrialized countries where excellent food control systems protect the consumer, food contamination, especially biological, remains an unquestionable risk.

Although there is clear knowledge (except in rare cases) on *what* to do to ensure nutrition while sustaining the environment, it is not always known *how* to implement the recommended measures. Though environmental problems are similar in different countries, their relative importance varies according to the respective conditions and geography (OECD, 1989).

## REFERENCES

ACC/SCN, United Nations (1989). Update on the nutrition situation: Recent trends in nutrition in 33 countries.

Allaway, W. H. (1986). Soil-plant-animal and human interrelationships in trace element nutrition. In: *Trace Elements in Human and Animal Nutrition*, **2**, 465–88, Academic Press.

American Association for the Advancement of Science, Sub-Saharan Africa Program (1991). Malaria and development in Africa: A cross-sectoral approach, Washington, D.C.

Arthur, J. R., Nicol, F., and Beckett, J. (1990). Hepatic iodothyronine 5′ deiodinase: The role of selenium. *Biochemical Journal*, **272**(2), 537–40.

Biswas, A. K. (1992). Freshwater environment, 1972–1992. *Water International*, **17**(2).

Biswas, A. K. (1991). Land and water development for sustainable agricultural development of Egypt: Opportunities and constraints. Report to Economic and Social Policy Division, FAO, Rome.

Biswas, A. K. (1990). Impacts of agriculture on water quality: A state-of-the-art review. Report to Water Management Division, FAO, Rome.

Biswas, A. K. (1987). Monitoring and evaluation of irrigated agriculture: A case study of Bhima Project, India. *Food Policy*, **12**(1), 47–61.

Biswas, A. K. and Arar, A. (1988). *Treatment and Reuse of Wastewater*, Butterworths, London, 186 pp.

Biswas, M. and Biswas, A. K. (1981). Interview with President Ziaur Rahman. *Mazingira*, **5**(3), 2–7.

Cleaver, K. and Schreiber, G. (1992). Population, agriculture and the environment in Africa. *Finance and Development*, June 1992.

Conway, G. R. and Pretty, J. N. (1990). Pollution and farming systems. International Symposium on Asian Farming Systems, Asian Institute of Technology, Bangkok, November 1990.

Economic Research Service (1990). China: Agriculture and trade report. *Situation and Outlook Series*, Report RS-90–3, U.S. Department of Agriculture, Washington, D.C., 37–40.

El-Hinnawi, E. (1991). Sustainable agriculture and rural development in the Near East. Regional Document No. 4, FAO/Netherlands Conference on Agriculture and Environment, FAO, Rome.

Esrey, S. A. and Feachem, R. G. (1989). Interventions for the control of diarrhoeal disease. Geneva Diarrhoeal Disease Control, WHO, unpublished.

FAO (1990). *The Conservation and Rehabilitation of African Lands*, FAO, Rome, 38 pp.

FAO (1978–1990). *FAO Production Yearbooks*, 1977–1989, FAO, Rome.

Gopalan, C. (1991). Challenges and frontiers in nutrition in Asia. Plenary Lecture, Sixth Asian Congress of Nutrition, Kuala Lumpur, Malaysia, 16–19 September 1991.

Greeley, M. (1987). *Post-harvest Losses, Technology and Employment: The Case of Rice in Bangladesh*, Westview Press, Boulder, 13–21.

Hardoy, J. E. and Satterthwaite, D. (1989). *Squatter Citizen: Life in the Urban Third World*, Earthscan Publications, London.

ICN (1992). Preventing specific micronutrient deficiencies. In: *Major Issues for Nutrition Strategies 1992*, Theme Paper No. 6, FAO, Rome and WHO, Geneva.

Igbedioh, S. O. (1992). Minimizing environmental and health effects of agricultural pesticides in developing countries. *Ambio*, **20**(6), September 1991, 219–21.

Igbedioh, S. O. and Akinyele, I. O. (1992). What future for food control in developing countries? Some lessons from Nigeria. *Ecology of Food and Nutrition*, **27**, 127–32.

Kanwar, J. S. (1990). Inaugural Address at Micronutrient Workshop, Andhra Pradesh Agricultural University, Andhra Pradesh, India.

Kenmore, P., Litsinger, J. A., Bandong, J. P., Santiago, A. C., and Salac, M. M. (1987). Philippine rice farmers and insecticides. In: Tait, E. J. and Napompeth, B. (eds), *Management of Pests and Pesticides: Farmers' Perceptions and Practices*, Westview Press, London.

Malaria Research Centre. *Bio-environmental Control of Malaria*, New Delhi.

Mannan, A. and Rahim, A. (eds) (1988). *Zinc in Nutrition*. Bangladesh Agricultural Research Council, Dacca.

Mill, A. (1992). Rodent control. *Far Eastern Agriculture*, May/June, 10–11.

Minister of Health, Morocco (1991). Personal communication, Rabat.

Nriagu, J. (1992). Toxic metal pollution in Africa. *The Science of the Total Environment*, **121**, 1–37.

OECD (1991). *The State of the Environment*, OECD, Paris, 295 pp.

OECD (1989). *Agricultural and Environmental Policies: Opportunities for Integration*, OECD, Paris, 82–83.

Parr *et al.* (1991). Minor and trace elements in human milk. *Biological Trace Element Research*, **29**, 51–75.

Pimentel, D. *et al.* (1991). Environmental and economic effects of reducing pesticide use. *BioScience*, **41**(6), 402–9.

Sharma, V. P. (1987). The Green Revolution in India and ecological succession of malaria vectors. 7th Annual Meeting, WHO/FAO/UNEP Panel of Experts on Environmental Management of Vector Control, 7–11 September, FAO, Rome.

Swaminathan, M. S. (1991). Agriculture and food production. Unpublished manuscript submitted to UNEP, Nairobi.

Swaminathan, M. S. (1991a). From Stockholm to Rio de Janeiro, Monograph No. 5, M.S. Swaminathan Research Foundation, Madras.

Tomatis, L. (ed.) (1990). *Cancer: Causes, Occurrence and Control*, International Agency for Research on Cancer, Lyon.

UNEP (1992). The status of desertification and implementation of UN Plan of Action to Combat Desertification, Nairobi.

UNEP (1992a). Chemical pollution: a global overview, Geneva, 5–18.

UNEP (1986). *The State of the Environment 1986: Environment and Health*, Nairobi.

UNEP/FAO/WHO (1988). Assessment of chemical contaminants in food. Report on the results of the UNEP/FAO/WHO Programme on Health-Related Environmental Monitoring, WHO, Geneva.

UNFPA (1992). *The State of World Population 1992*, New York, 46 pp.

UNICEF (1989). *The State of the World's Children 1989*, Oxford, Oxford University Press.

WHO (1992). *Our Planet, Our Health, Report of the WHO Commission on Health and Environment*, Geneva, 1–144.

WHO (1990). The impact of development policies on health: Review of the literature, Geneva.

WHO (1984). The role of food safety in health and development. Report of a Joint FAO/WHO Expert Committee on Food Safety. WHO Technical Report Series, No. 705, Geneva.

WHO (1978). *Nitrates, nitrites and N-nitrose compounds*. WHO Environmental Health Criteria, No. 5, Geneva.

World Bank (1992). *World Development Report 1992: Development and the Environment*, Oxford, Oxford University Press.

World Resources Institute (1990). *World Resources 1990–91*, Oxford, Oxford University Press.

Zaidi *et al.* (1989). Trends in ambient levels of DDT and HCH residues in humans and the environment of Delhi, India. In: Nair, A. and Pillai, M. K. (eds) (1992), *The Science of the Total Environment*, **121**, 145–57.

# 2

# Trends in Food Consumption Patterns: Impact of developmental transition

## C. GOPALAN

## INTRODUCTION

The food-consumption patterns of populations are broadly governed by two sets of factors, namely:

1. the range of foods, either locally produced or imported, available in a region and in a given season, which are within the people's actual physical and economic reach, and
2. cultural practices (belief-systems, tastes, prejudices, fads, and taboos) and traditional customs which influence the actual choice and mix of such foods.

Generally speaking, for several centuries now—indeed till almost the middle of the current century—there had been no remarkable changes in the range of naturally-occurring foods, nor any major shifts in food-consumption patterns in different regions of the world. During the last few decades, however, man's food-consumption patterns have been undergoing significant changes, and the health consequences of such changes—both beneficial and deleterious—are becoming increasingly manifest. Leaving aside a historical review of food-consumption patterns down through the ages, and confining the discussion to changes in food-consumption patterns induced by socio-economic developmental transition during recent decades, we proceed to briefly consider the health consequences of such changes.

## FACTORS CONTRIBUTING TO RECENT CHANGES IN FOOD-CONSUMPTION PATTERNS

The major factors contributing to changing food-consumption patterns in recent decades are now elucidated.

### New Agricultural and Food Technologies

Notable advances in agricultural and food technologies during the last four decades have, on the one hand, augmented the overall availability of certain foods (e.g. wheat and rice in some parts of the world). This has been a major beneficial contribution, especially for those countries whose populations subsist on predominantly cereal-based diets. On the other hand, the Green Revolution, because of its near-exclusive emphasis on wheat and rice, has indirectly contributed to a distortion of the pattern of relative availability of food grains, and a decline in the per caput availability of pulses and legumes. The result is that pulses are now beyond the economic reach of the poorest sections of populations in developing countries, resulting in the deterioration of the protein quality of diets in these poverty-stricken households.

Improved methods of storage and preservation (especially of perishables), modernized culinary techniques, and newer methods of food processing have contributed to increased availability of 'convenience (ready-to-eat) foods', and consequent changes in dietary mores, especially in urban and semi-urban areas. Commercial infant foods are a striking example of a product of modern food technology that has had a profound impact (unfortunately, largely deleterious in this case) on the salutary practice of breast-feeding. The growing popularity of commercial baby foods in early infancy in urban slums of the developing countries is resulting in harmful repercussions on the health of infants and children.

### Improvements in Food Distribution and Marketing Systems

Well-coordinated marketing management has facilitated a wider choice of foods and provided incentives to increased production; more importantly, in the case of several developing countries, especially those of South Asia, such updated techniques have contributed also to the near-eradication of recurrent acute famines, which used to devastate populations in pockets of poverty during scarcity seasons, and to controlling wide seasonal fluctuations in food-consumption patterns. Early warning systems, and better facilities for rapid transport of foods to distress areas, have promoted greater food and nutrition security.

## Scientific and Technological Advances Outside the Fields of Food and Agriculture

Scientific advances in such fields as industry, electronics, biotechnology, information, and transport have brought about marked changes in occupational patterns of both men and women; family structures; living styles; and value systems of population groups. These transformations are being inevitably reflected in food-consumption patterns.

## Large-scale Migration of Rural Populations to Urban Areas

Mass human transfers from rural to urban zones have induced changes in food-consumption patterns, and infant-feeding and child-rearing practices, especially among large numbers of slum populations in urban areas in several developing countries. This migration has been necessitated, on the one hand, by the induction of a wide array of labour-saving devices, and the displacement of the marginal landholder in the wake of the new agricultural technology; and, on the other hand, by rapid industrialization which offers expanding job opportunities for displaced agricultural labour (both men and women) in urban and semi-urban areas.

## Rising Income Levels

Income levels are a major determinant of the degree of a population's access to food and of the nature of their choice of foods. Large sections of mankind in poor developing countries continue to live below the poverty line and are unable to secure food of adequate quantity and good quality. The speed of change in their food-consumption patterns will depend directly on the pace at which their poverty is alleviated and their incomes rise to levels permitting adequate access to food.

On the other hand, all over the world including the developing countries, sizeable numbers of people have not only overcome poverty but have even reached the rungs of affluence where food is easily accessible. Some of those who have thus succeeded are the neo-rich. Epidemiological studies would suggest that it is this section of the population that is most prone to dietary excesses and errors, and therefore most vulnerable to consequent health hazards.

## Scientific Advances in Nutrition Science

In recent years, scientific advances have promoted the understanding of the right choice of foods for the promotion and preservation of health and physical fitness. Nutrition education, based on such sound scientific knowledge, is playing a significant role in bringing about beneficial changes in food-consumption patterns; and these have already resulted in arresting earlier disturbing escalations of some degenerative diseases (e.g. reduction in the incidence of coronary heart disease with reduction in dietary fat intake) observed in some affluent societies. They have also been instrumental in overcoming problems of ill-health related to under-nutrition and specific nutrient deficiencies in several developing countries. However, a good part of what passes for 'nutrition education' is, unfortunately, not based on science, but quackery, and tends to promote faulty dietary practices. This masquerade needs to be unveiled and corrected.

Currently, societies in most parts of the world are, as it were, in a state of 'transition' induced by economic, social, and political forces on the one side, and by scientific and technological progress on the other. The pace of this transition varies from country-to-country and, within each country, from community-to-community. Many of the factors briefly discussed above are operating to varying extents in most of these societies.

Depending on the stage of 'development' of a country and the speed of its transition process, changes in food-consumption patterns may vary both with respect to their nature and degree. Experience from developing countries in a state of dynamic developmental transition, and comparative studies of the rich and poor sections within such countries, may prove particularly illuminating. We shall therefore briefly consider changing food-consumption patterns in both the so-called 'developing' and 'developed' countries. The latter (the 'First World') is largely formed by an affluent society which permits unlimited access to foods of choice. The former category (the 'Third World'), on the other hand, is composed of peoples who represent both ends of the socio-economic spectrum: while large sections of the population are still below the poverty line, sizeable numbers are throwing off the shackles of poverty, and some have even attained affluence and freedom from economic constraints on their access to, and choice of, foods.

## DEVELOPING COUNTRIES

### Food-consumption Patterns among the Rural Poor (Low-income Groups)

Our observations on food-consumption patterns of the rural poor are based largely on experience in India and, to a certain extent, in other South East Asian countries, but they may be generally applicable to most developing countries.

A major boost to foodgrain (wheat and rice) production in Asia, as in many other parts of the world during the last three decades, was provided by the introduction of the new agricultural technology, which is based on high-yielding seed varieties and intensified use of chemical fertilizers. It is evident that this development led to the remarkable augmentation of overall cereal production and helped the agricultural nations to belie the alarming and gloomy prophecies of the late sixties. For example, thanks to the Green Revolution, India's overall foodgrain production rose from 62.7 million tonnes in 1956 to 138.41 million tonnes by 1990, and the per caput availability of foodgrains had not declined despite the phenomenal growth of population in the intervening years. However, the Green Revolution had its own limitations:

1. the near-neglect of pulses and legumes, resulting in significant decline in per caput availability of pulses from 61 g/day in 1951 to 33 g/day in 1988;
2. relative neglect of millets, leading to a decrease in their overall production;
3. no significant gains in respect of production of vegetables and fruits;
4. progressive depletion of soil micronutrients because of excessive use of chemical fertilizers, and excessive irrigation leading to salinity and alkalinization of soils.

These limitations, along with the fact that there were no major parallel socio-economic initiatives towards achieving equitable food distribution through narrowing of gross disparities in income levels of population groups, resulted in a situation wherein, while acute starvation and large-scale famines in the countries of the Indian subcontinent were avoided, diets in the lowest income groups of their populations continue

**Table 2.1** Average consumption of foodstuffs (g/CU/day) in rural low-income groups in India

| Foodstuffs | 1975–79 | 1988–90 |
|---|---|---|
| Cereals and millets | 504 | 490 |
| Pulses | 36 | 32 |
| Green, leafy vegetables | 8 | 11 |
| Other vegetables | 51 | 49 |
| Roots and tubers | 48 | 40 |
| Milk and milk products | 100 | 96 |
| Fats and oils | 12 | 13 |
| Sugar and jaggery | 23 | 29 |

Source: NNMB, Report on Repeat Surveys (1988–90), NIN, ICMR, 1991

to be deficient in quantity and quality. A typical diet of low-income group households in India (Table 2.1) will highlight this point.

It must, however, be pointed out that, though 'average' diets among the poor do not reflect any major improvement during the last few decades, disaggregated data from within the low-income groups reveal that the proportion of poor in the *lowest* income brackets within the low-income group has significantly dwindled. In short, abject poverty is on the wane; and, as a result, the prevalence of florid nutritional deficiency diseases has declined. Thus, severe malnutrition in children in India had dropped from 15 per cent in 1975–79 to 8.7 per cent in 1988–90 (National Nutrition Monitoring Bureau, 1991), for the reason that most cases of severe malnutrition are drawn from the *lowest* income brackets (the abjectly poor) in the low-income category.

Disaggregated data from low-, middle-, and high-income groups throw light on the effect of rising income levels on food-consumption patterns in populations slowly overcoming poverty. The striking differences in food-consumption patterns in India, as between the higher income groups on the one hand and the urban slum-dwellers and the rural poor on the other, are evident in the data in Table 2.2. These wide disparities in food-consumption patterns are reflected in the anthropometric status of both children and adults, as also in the profile of diseases to which they are subject (see Table 2.3, and Figs. 2.1 and 2.2).

## Fat Intake in the Affluent

Currently, there are distinct differences in the dietary intake of fat in populations of developing countries emerging from poverty. Thus, while

**Table 2.2** Comparative average consumption of foodstuffs (g/CU/day) (1975–79, India)

| Foodstuffs | Urban population | | Rural poor |
| | High income group | Slum dwellers | |
| --- | --- | --- | --- |
| Cereals and millets | 316 | 416 | 504 |
| Pulses | 57 | 33 | 36 |
| Green, leafy vegetables | 21 | 11 | 8 |
| Other vegetables | 113 | 40 | 51 |
| Roots and tubers | 82 | 70 | 48 |
| Milk | 424 | 42 | 100 |
| Fats and oils | 46 | 13 | 12 |
| Sugar and jaggery | 34 | 20 | 23 |

Sources: NNMB, Report on Repeat Surveys (1988–90), NIN, ICMR, 1991. NNMB, Report on Urban Population (1975–79) NIN, ICMR, 1984

**Table 2.3** Average weights and heights of adults (20–25 years)

| Income group | Male | | Female | |
| | Height (cm) | Weight (kg) | Height (cm) | Weight (kg) |
| --- | --- | --- | --- | --- |
| Urban | | | | |
| High income | 166.4 | 50.4 | 154.6 | 46.8 |
| Slum dwellers | 161.4 | 46.6 | 150.1 | 41.7 |
| Rural poor | 163.1 | 48.2 | 150.9 | 42.7 |

Sources: NNMB, Report on Repeat Surveys (1988–90), NIN, ICMR, 1991. NNMB, Report on Urban Population (1975–79) NIN, ICMR, 1984.

the diets of 17 per cent of Indian households made up of the poorest income-groups do not include any visible fat (as against 'invisible' fat present in cereals and pulses), it could be computed that 5 per cent of India's population, largely composed of the urban rich, consume nearly 40 per cent of all the fat available in the country. This works out roughly to a per caput availability of the order of 125–130 g fat daily for the affluent. Allowing for the inevitable wastes, fat consumption (accounted for by 'visible' fat) could easily account for over 30 per cent of total calories in the diets of the most affluent sections.

Fat intake by the well-to-do as compared with that of the poor varies not only in respect of quantity but also in respect of the type of fat

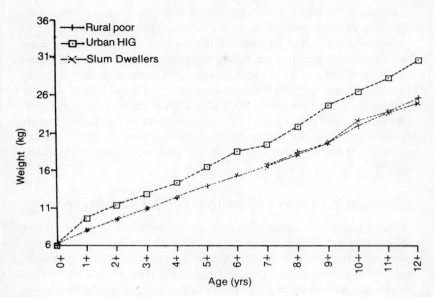

**Fig. 2.1**  Average weights of boys

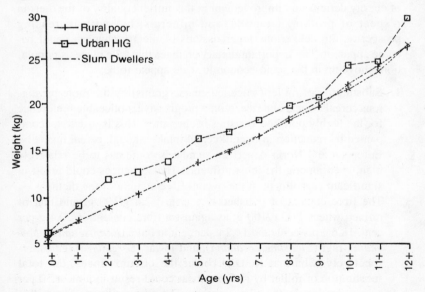

**Fig. 2.2**  Average weights of girls

consumed. Fat intake in the dietaries of the affluent includes high proportions of hydrogenated vegetable fat and ghee (clarified butter). In computing the overall fat intake in the dietaries of the affluent, it must also be remembered that practically every food item in traditional Indian diets (based on cereals and legumes) contains some fat as 'invisible' fat. Such 'invisible' fat in the diet could account for an additional 20 g fat intake daily, but fortunately much of this fat is made up of 'beneficial' polyunsaturated fatty acids. Thus, the overall fat intake in the most affluent sections of the population of even developing countries such as India must be considered as excessive and not conducive to sound health.

## Changes in Dietary Pattern Induced by 'Development'

Piecing together evidence from numerous diet surveys among different population segments in developing countries in varying stages of transition, we may conclude that emergence from poverty, urban migration, and socio-economic advancement bring about changes not only in lifestyles but also in dietary patterns of populations. The changes in the initial phases of development may be beneficial, resulting in correction of energy deficits and improvement in the nutrient quality of the diets in respect of protein, vitamins, and minerals; but with increasing prosperity, the deleterious repercussions of dietary changes could become apparent. The important dietary changes that take place as populations move up in the socio-economic scale appear to be:

1. Substitution of millet (so-called coarse grains) by the more prestigious cereals wheat and rice, with a progressive, noticeable preference for the highly polished varieties of the latter. This is usually accompanied by reduction in overall cereal intake (though cereal intake by European and North American standards continues to be relatively high, even among the most affluent). These changes could result in significant curtailment in the overall fibre content of the diet.
   The fibre content of polished rice is just 2.4 g/100 g, and that of refined wheat 3.00 g/100 g, as against a fibre content of 20.4 g per cent, 18.6 g per cent, and 14.2 g per cent in bajra (*Pennisetum typhoideum*), ragi (*Eleusime coracana*), and jowar (*Sorghum vulgare*), respectively (Sharma, R. D.). Under the circumstances, the total substitution of millet by rice or wheat could result in almost 50 per cent reduction in the fibre content. The fibre content of raw rice

**Table 2.4** Fibre content of Indian foods

| | |
|---|---|
| Millets | |
| Bajra (*Penniscum typhoideum*) | 20.4 g% |
| Jowar (*Sorghum vulgare*) | 14.2 g% |
| Maize (*Zea mays*) | 6.8 g% |
| Ragi (*Eleusime coracana*) | 18.6 g% |
| Wheat | |
| Wholemeal (100%) | 9.6 g% |
| Refined | 3.0 g% |
| Rice | |
| Raw (brown) | 5–8 g% |
| Polished | 2.4 g% |

Chemical Nature of Cereal Fibre

| | |
|---|---|
| Non-celluloid polysacharide | 48.9–61.5 % |
| Celluloid | 31.8–32.7% |
| Liguin | 6.7–18.4% |

Estimated Total Fibre Content of Average Indian Cereal-based Dietaries

| | |
|---|---|
| Wheat-based | 57.7 g/day/person |
| Rice-based | 33.2 g/day/person |
| Millet-based | 90.0 g/day/person |

Source: R. D. Sharma, National Institute of Nutrition, Personal Communication

(brown) is 5–8 g/100 g as against 2.4 g/100 g for polished rice; the fibre content of wholemeal wheat (100 per cent) is 9.6 g/100 g as against 3.0 g/100 g for refined wheat (Table 2.4).

2. Increased consumption of legumes, vegetables, and milk, which may be considered beneficial changes.
3. Continued low intake of green, leafy vegetables, which are perhaps scorned as the 'poor man's food'; hence their low social prestige. The fact that is overlooked is that green, leafy vegetables are not only a rich source of carotene, folic acid, vitamin C, and calcium but also of linoleic acid.
4. Progressive increase in fat intake, with a growing preference for hydrogenated fat in place of vegetable oils (in the case of the middle classes), and a relatively high intake of ghee, i.e. clarified butter, among the most prosperous sections.
5. Higher intake of sugar.

6. Increase in overall energy absorption in relation to energy expenditure.

## HEALTH CONSEQUENCES OF CHANGES IN FOOD-CONSUMPTION PATTERNS IN DEVELOPING COUNTRIES

### Low-income Group

Improvements in the diets of the poorest sections of mankind have already resulted in the progressive reduction and near-elimination of florid, nutritional-deficiency diseases that used to afflict the developing countries until a few decades ago. The virtual disappearance of beri beri (cardiac and dry types) from large parts of Asia; the subsidence of pellagra from the Deccan plateau of India, and the countries bordering the Mediterranean and southern United States; a steep decline in the incidence of keratomalacia from parts of north India, Pakistan, Bangladesh, and Indonesia; a lower incidence of goitre over large parts of the world; the subsidence of osteomalacia from parts of north India and Pakistan—all these are 'success stories'. Kwashiorkor of the classical 'blubbery' type with crazy-pavement dermatosis and huge fatty livers has already passed into history, and what has now taken its place is so-called 'moderate' and 'severe malnutrition', identified largely by the degree of growth-retardation rather than by glaring clinical signs. All these successes are not perhaps solely attributable to changing food consumption patterns alone, but also to concomitant control of infections and better preventive health services and specific technological interventions (for instance, iodization of common salt in the case of goitre).

### Urban Slums

Rapid urbanization and the expanding urban slum population will perhaps pose the greatest challenge to developing countries in the next two decades. Nearly a third of the population of South East Asia will be urban by AD 2000, and a third of these urban dwellers will be living in slums. The urban slum population in India alone is thus expected to exceed 100 million by AD 2000. Women living in the slums will be compelled to seek employment opportunities outside their homes—in factories and in the informal sectors—to supplement the family income. This will pose a serious threat to the current salutary practice of breast-feeding. Indeed, the entire pattern of diets in infancy and childhood in urban slum-dwellers will be revolutionized. Attention to the increasing unhygienic use of commercial baby foods in urban slums had already been drawn in an earlier communication (Gopujkar, P. V. *et al.*, 1984). Unhygienic ready-to-eat foods are sure to multiply the number of infections which are already undermining infant and child health in these countries.

Currently, most of the 'street foods' sold in the urban slums of Asia are based on traditional food items and are generally served fresh and hot, but this could change if 'inexpensive' imitations of fashionable non-traditional 'fast foods' take their place. Salmonellosis, and other types of food contamination in such cheap fast foods, could pose problems. Such unhealthy foods could also enter into the dietaries of children, with obvious harmful reactions. Imaginative initiatives will therefore be needed to contain and counter these disturbing emerging trends.

## High-income Group

The transformation in food-consumption patterns brought about by affluence is apparently contributing to the revolution in respect of the prevalence of such degenerative maladies as coronary heart disease and diabetes (Type II) in several developing countries. (See also chapter 8).

### Coronary heart diseases

Chadha and colleagues (1990) in India found that the prevalence of coronary heart disease (CHD) in urban Delhi was over six times (7.3 per cent) that in its rural environment, and that the victims were largely drawn from the most affluent sections of the population. Studies in Britain had demonstrated that Indian immigrants in Britain had a higher morbidity and standardized mortality ratio for CHD than the indigenous population. Jacobson (1987) had attributed the higher morbidity and mortality from CHD of Indian immigrants in Britain to the consumption of ghee, a clarified butter product which, unlike fresh butter, was found to contain substantial amounts of cholesterol oxides. Miller *et al.* (1984) observed that Indian immigrants had relatively low levels of HDL cholesterol and lower proportions of polyunsaturated fatty acids (PUFA) as omega-3 fatty acids—biochemical findings indicative of increased susceptibility to coronary heart disease.

### Diabetes

Mather and Keen (1985) have shown that the prevalence of diabetes

(Type II) in Indian immigrants in London was nearly 3.8 times that among Europeans of all age groups; the difference was nearly five-fold when only the 40–50 year age group was considered. The incidence of diabetes among Indians immigrants in London corresponded closely to the prevalence rate among affluent Indians in Delhi, using the same investigative parameters (Verma *et al.*, 1986). On the other hand, an earlier ICMR study had revealed that the prevalence of diabetes among the rural poor was only half that in the urban population (1.1 per cent as against 2.2 per cent). An investigation in Singapore covering Indians, Malays, and Chinese (Thai *et al.*, 1987) showed that the prevalence of diabetes was decidedly higher than that observed in the same population group 15 years earlier.

## Hypertension

Miller *et al.* (1984) had also reported that the prevalence of hypertension among immigrant Indians in Britain was as high as 40 per cent, as against 20–25 per cent in European and West-Indians in that country. Indian diets generally contain high concentrations of salt, spices, and condiments.

These observations indicate that, unlike in the case of the poor, the problems posed by the rising incidence of degenerative diseases could be at least as serious (if not more so) among the affluent populations of developing countries as among those of industrialized countries. Epidemiological studies show that even modest advances in prosperity in populations with low GNP are associated with most marked increases in the incidence of degenerative disease. The data on the affluent sections of India's population and on Indian migrants to Britain referred to above will illustrate this point. Affluent Indians, either in India or in London, are by no means more prosperous than the affluent sections of their countries of adoption, but the fact that they appear more prone to degenerative diseases may be the result of the more rapid transition (intra-generational) in their food-consumption patterns.

As stated earlier, most of the data on developing countries presented above are based on the Indian experience, but they are largely applicable to several other countries in 'developmental transition'. The data contained in the exhaustive report on *Diet, nutrition and the prevention of chronic disease* by WHO (1990) would justify such a conclusion.

## Comparison of overall food-consumption patterns in developing and developed countries

The impact of rising affluence on food-consumption patterns is strikingly evident in the data on overall per caput food supply and food consumption in countries in different stages of developmental transition. It is clear from the figures in Table 2.5 that while levels of food supply and per caput daily protein intake are marginally adequate in the relatively poor countries, they far exceed generally-accepted nutritional requirements in highly affluent societies. The data on daily meat consumption highlight this difference most strikingly (Table 2.6).

**Table 2.5** Food supply patterns in selected countries in 1988 (per caput/day)

| Countries | Calories (kcal) | Proteins (g) | Fat (g) |
| --- | --- | --- | --- |
| USA | 3666 | 109.3 | 163.8 |
| Argentina | 3118 | 102.6 | 106.8 |
| Japan | 2848 | 90.8 | 82.1 |
| Brazil | 2709 | 62.6 | 64.3 |
| China | 2632 | 63.4 | 43.7 |
| Colombia | 2561 | 56.5 | 56.5 |
| Zimbabwe | 2312 | 57.5 | 57.7 |
| Nigeria | 2062 | 48.8 | 40.9 |
| India[*] | 2008–2603 | 53.4–73.1 | 13–46 |

Source: FAO, Food Balance Sheets, FAO, Rome 1991
[*]NNMB, Report on Urban Population (1975–79), NIN, ICMR 1984

**Table 2.6** Meat supply per capita

| Countries | g/day |
| --- | --- |
| USA | 305.9 |
| Argentina | 286.4 |
| Japan | 91.4 |
| Colombia | 84.4 |
| Brazil | 79.6 |
| China | 51.5 |
| Zimbabwe | 31.6 |
| Nigeria | 24.4 |
| India[*] | <31 |

Source: FAO, Food Balance Sheets, FAO, Rome 1991
[*]NNMB, Report on Urban Population (1975–79), NIN, ICMR 1984

Incidentally, while a great deal of concern is often expressed over excessive fat intake in affluent populations, because of the increased hazards of degenerative heart diseases attributable to such excessive fat intake, there is hardly any censure of the needlessly high, almost wasteful, levels of consumption of animal proteins in some affluent societies, far in excess of human physiological requirements even by the most generous standards. Harmful effects of excessive intakes of animal proteins have not yet been identified, though there is suggestive evidence that the very high incidence of osteoporosis and fractures of the neck of the femur in some affluent countries (despite a seemingly high intake of calcium) in contrast to the low incidence of that condition among poor populations (subsisting on lower calcium levels) could be possibly attributed to the obligatory loss of calcium induced by high protein diets. Nutrition education directed to discourage excessive meat consumption is eminently relevant in some affluent population groups.

As may be expected, the wide disparities in the food-consumption pattern of 'developed' and 'developing' countries is strikingly reflected in the reported causes of deaths of their respective populations (Table 2.7). Degenerative heart diseases and neoplasms account for over 70 per cent of all deaths in developed countries as against less than 25 per cent in developing countries. On the other hand, while infections and parasitic diseases and perinatal mortality, together accounted for barely 10 per cent of all deaths in developed countries, they accounted for nearly 50 per cent of all deaths in developing countries.

In assessing the impact of changes in food-consumption patterns on the profile of diseases, however, it must be recognized that such changes are always accompanied by parallel changes in socio-economic status,

**Table 2.7** Cause of death in 1980

| Causes of death | Percentage of deaths | |
| --- | --- | --- |
| | Developed countries | Developing countries |
| Diseases of the circulatory system | 54 | 19 |
| Neoplasms | 19 | 5 |
| Infectious and parasitic diseases | 8 | 40 |
| Injury and poisoning | 6 | 5 |
| Perinatal mortality | 2 | 8 |
| All other causes | 12 | 23 |

Source: WHO, Technical Report Series 797

lifestyles, occupational patterns, and environmental conditions. Under the circumstances, it is difficult to estimate, with precision, the role of dietary revision in the changing disease profile. Even so, it may be claimed that a revolutionized diet plays a more direct role in altering the disease profile for the reason that the other parallel factors mentioned often act by contributing to and facilitating dietary changes.

## HEALTH CONSEQUENCES OF CHANGES IN FOOD-CONSUMPTION PATTERNS IN DEVELOPED COUNTRIES

Advances in nutrition science, and increasing health/diet consciousness of populations, have facilitated some salutary changes in food-consumption patterns which have had beneficial impacts on the nutritional/health status. A few examples may be cited. The most outstanding is the return to breast-feeding in many affluent countries which had earlier almost completely substituted breast-feeding with artificial feeding. The nutritional superiority of breast milk over commercial baby foods has now been clearly established.

A steep reduction of over 40 per cent in the death rate from coronary heart diseases (CHD) in USA, Australia, and New Zealand is a noteworthy record. However, dietary changes alone have not wrought this transformation. It is estimated that 40 per cent of the recorded reduction could be due to more efficient, modern, medical intervention, a quarter to reduction in smoking, and about 30 per cent to changes in food-consumption patterns characterized by lower levels of fat intake (relatively higher intake of lean meat, low fat milk, and vegetable oils) and, particularly, a diminished consumption of foods rich in saturated fat. The downward trend in CHD witnessed in the USA has not been equally marked in some other affluent countries such as the UK, Finland, and Ireland. Ever since the classical 'seven country study', which served to highlight the impact of dietary factors and lifestyles on the incidence of CHD, there have been conscious efforts to discourage excessive fat intake, and these have been pursued more vigorously and effectively in countries such as USA and Australia than elsewhere.

## Cancers

An analysis of epidemiological data reveals that 20–30 per cent of cancers in men and 60 per cent in women are attributable to dietary factors.

Stomach cancer, which was among the leading causes of death in the USA in 1930, currently has about the lowest incidence rate in the world. In Japan also, stomach cancers which had a high rate of mortality have registered a gradual decline in recent years. This has been attributed to a decreased consumption of smoked and salt-preserved foods, which may be expected to contain a precursor of nitrosamines.

Several studies have traced the cause of breast cancers to excessive intake of saturated fats. But undisputed declines in its incidence, such as achieved in the elimination of CHD in the USA, have not been apparent in many affluent population groups.

Reductions in the incidence of ano-rectal cancers are being reported following successful movements directed to the promotion of higher intake of dietary fibre. Similarly, the beneficial effects of carotene-rich foods in the prevention and control of lung cancers are being increasingly recognized. This has led to emphasis on the advantages of a diet well-supplied with green and yellow vegetables rich in β-carotene.

## VEGETARIANISM AND OTHER RECENT TRENDS

### The Indian Scene

A high proportion of Indians are vegetarians, either because of traditional persuasions or economic reasons. Even non-vegetarian Indians do not eat meat daily; in any case, meat consumption in India, even in affluent households, is nowhere near the levels prevailing in those of Europe and North America. Among meats, beef is largely avoided by the Hindus (who constitute the predominant majority) and pork by the Muslims. Chicken, mutton, and fish are the usual non-vegetarian fare, the last being especially favoured in the eastern part of the country (Bengal). In general, it may be said that these traditional dietary patterns have not undergone radical changes under the impact of 'modernization'. Economic compulsions have in fact served to reinforce traditional vegetarianism. Milk and milk products have always been highly-valued food items in India, even among vegetarians. Ensuring protein quality in such 'lacto-vegetarian' dietaries has therefore posed no problem to nutrition scientists and dieticians.

Indian dietaries continue to be predominantly cereal-based; and this is unlikely to change significantly within the next few decades. The rigid, traditional, intraregional, and interregional preferences to chosen cereals (such as rice and wheat) among Indian populations have gradually weakened—a welcome development. The east and the south of the country were always the traditional 'rice belts', while the people of the north and the west were largely wheat consumers. The poor segments of the population in both north and south depended on millets as their main staple. In recent years, however, wheat is gaining popularity in south Indian dietaries, while rice consumption in the north and the west has also increased. When the poor ascend the socio-economic scale, they generally tend to discard millets in favour of the more prestigious rice and wheat—an option not particularly beneficial from the nutritional point of view, but which is being 'abetted', apart from social factors, by the relative neglect of millets during the years of the Green Revolution.

'Modernization', unfortunately, appears to have extracted its price in many ways. Some salutary traditional practices of food processing and cooking, earlier in vogue in India, are now increasingly being over-looked. Thus, the traditional practice of hand-pounding, which results in a cereal of good nutritive value, has largely given place to polishing and milling. Highly-polished 'white' rice is preferred by the affluent and therefore enjoys social prestige among the poor. It is more expensive and of poorer nutritive value! Traditional, simple household methods of 'malting' of cereals and 'sprouting' of grams, which significantly en-hance the digestibility and nutritive value of cereals and pulses, are no longer being widely practised. Amylase-rich malted cereals, which dis-tinctly enhance the calorie density of cereal-based weaning dietaries, could have been used to combat the 'bulk factor' (low calorie density), which is the major hurdle in ensuring adequacy of calorie intake in later infancy and early childhood. The younger generation of the middle-class and affluent income groups is increasingly partial to 'soft drinks'. Also, 'convenience foods' and 'fast foods' are slowly becoming fashionable fare, especially in urban and semi-urban areas; but, currently, there is no adequate infrastructure which could ensure the wholesomeness of these foods.

## The General Global Pattern

Recent years have brought increasing recognition of the 'virtues of vegetarianism', even in the industrialized countries of Europe and North America. Vegetarianism seems to be gaining scientific 'respectability' instead of remaining in its customary 'cult' niche. A growing awareness of the qualities in vegetable ingredients that 'protect and promote health' is revolutionizing food preferences. The importance of fibre (a significant component of cereal-based diets), originally dismissed as 'roughage', is now better understood. There is also increasing conviction of the benefits of vegetable foods in respect of prevention and management of degenerative diseases, though hard scientific data in this area are not easily available. The newly-discovered protective role of carotenoids in some forms of cancer (especially lung cancer) has served to underscore the importance of green, leafy vegetables. Some vegetable foods are also known to be good sources of omega-3 fatty acids, the importance of which in ensuring proper fatty-acid balance in the diet is now established. The so-called 'invisible fats' of cereals are fair sources of 'desirable' fatty acids.

Even among animal (non-vegetarian) foods, updated nutrition knowledge has led to a growing preference for lean meat and fish. There is not only a movement away from excessive consumption of fats, but also a recognition of the need to ensure a right mix of fatty acids in the diet. This has led to increasing appreciation of the nutritive value of such foods as fish and vegetables.

Crusading for moderation in alcohol consumption has also gained ground, following on the realization of the deleterious effects of excess alcohol consumption on coronary heart diseases and colonic cancer.

There is growing consciousness among the young and the old of the need for avoiding obesity; in particular, the deleterious implications of central ('apple') obesity have been widely publicized. Slimming exercises and slimming diets are more consciously practised now than in the past, both in developed and developing countries. Indeed, 'slimming industries' are flourishing in all big and small cities of the world, though the dietary regimes that these sometimes advocate for speedy, spectacular results may not stand scientific scrutiny. There is increasing health (and weight) consciousness among the younger generation, though this may not always be actually reflected in the correct choice of foods. On the whole, there is apparently far greater scope and opportunity now for *successful* nutrition education, and inculcation of dietary discipline, than ever before. All these features are welcome trends in food-consumption patterns.

## CONCLUSIONS

It is obvious that both deficiencies and excesses in respect of food consumption could exert deleterious health consequences, as has been diagrammatically indicated in Fig. 2.3. National nutrition policies must

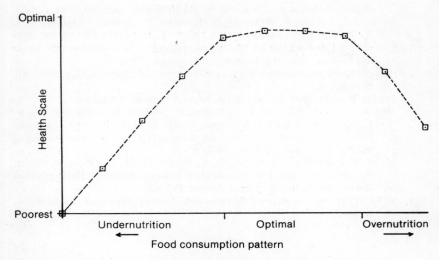

**Fig. 2.3** Health consequences of changing food-consumption patterns

ensure that the food-consumption patterns are such as to maintain mankind in the optimal state of health. This goal can be achieved if diets are in balance, i.e. neither deficient nor in excess. Equally essential is the need for promotion of proper dietary guidelines for populations in different levels of socio-economic development and currently subsisting on different patterns of food consumption—a task that is particularly challenging in the case of developing countries wherein both ends of the food-consumption spectrum (deficiency and excess) are represented.

## REFERENCES

Chadha, S. L., Radhakrishnan, S., Ramachandran, K., Kaul, U., and Gopinath, N. (1990). Epidemiological study of coronary heart disease in urban population of Delhi. *Indian Journal of Medical Res*earch [B], **92**, 424–30.

Gopujkar, P. V., Chaudhuri, S. N., Ramaswami, M. A., Gore, M. S., and Gopalan, C. (1984). Infant feeding practices with special references to the use of commercial infant foods. Scientific Report 4, Nutrition Foundation of India.

Jacobson, M. D. (1987). Cholesterol oxides in Indian ghee: Possible cause of unexplained high risk of artheroclerosis in Indian immigrant population. *Lancet*, **2**, 656–8.

## 54 / C. Gopalan

Mather, H. M. and Keen, H. (1985). The Southall diabetes survey: Prevalence of diabetes in Asians and Europeans. *British Medical Journal*, **291**, 1081.

Miller, G. J., Kotecha, S., Wilkinson, W. H., Wilkes, H., Sterling, Y., Sanders, T. A. B., Brodherst, A., Alison, J., and Meade, T. W. (1984). Dietary and other characteristics relevant for coronary heart disease in men of India, West Indian and European descent in London. *Atherosclerosis*, **70**, 63–72.

National Nutrition Monitoring Bureau (1991). Report of Repeat Surveys (1988–90), NIN, ICMR.

Sharma, R. D. Personal communication, National Institute of Nutrition.

Thai, A. C., Yeo, P. P. B., Lun, K. C., Hughes, K., Wang, K. W., Sothy, S. P., Lui, K. F., Ng, W. Y., Cheah, J. S., Phoon, W. O., and Lim, P. (1987). Changing prevalence of diabetes mellitus in Singapore over a ten-year period. *Journal of Medical Association, Thailand*, **70**(2), 63–7.

Verma, N. P. S., Mehta, S. P., Madhu, S., Mather, H. M., and Keen, H. (1986). Prevalence of known diabetes in an urban Indian environment: The Darya Ganj diabetes survey. *British Medical Journal*, **293**, 423.

WHO (1990). Diet, nutrition and the prevention of chronic diseases. *Technical Report Series*, 797.

# 3

# Food Security and Poor Urban Populations

SARAH J. ATKINSON

## INTRODUCTION

The paucity of studies on urban nutrition and the bias towards rural problems has been highlighted over the last decade, and a core of papers reviewing issues in urban nutrition have sought to rectify this balance over recent years (Gross and Solomons, 1985; Schurch and Favre, 1985; Wray, 1986; Solomons and Gross, 1987; Viteri, 1987; Popkin and Bisgrove, 1987; Hussain and Lunven, 1987; Gross and Monteiro, 1989; Pryer, 1990; Atkinson, 1992). The argument for focusing more on urban nutrition than has been the case historically is that the urban population, particularly the poorer sections, is growing disproportionately fast (Donahue, 1982). In addition, the relative increase of the poor urban population represents, in part, a shift of the rural poor to the urban centres (Gilbert and Gugler, 1981). The World Bank (1991) has predicted that urban poverty will be the most vital development issue of the next century.

There are neither sufficient data on trends in malnutrition rates nor models predicting future trends in the absence of preventive measures for improvement of food security. One study along these lines has indicated the deteriorating status of health and nutrition in Thailand (Khanjanasthiti and Wray, 1974). Health statistics in countries said to be in transition, or post-transition, have indicated the increasing importance of chronic degenerative diseases, such as cardiovascular disease, many of which have food habits as an important risk factor. The idea that chronic diseases will be limited to the urban elite is not supported, and the poor are fast being subjected to risk from both types of disease patterns (Briscoe, 1989). The urban poor have been said to suffer the worst of both worlds (Harpham *et al.*, 1988).

The crucial goal for planners of food policy is the provision of adequate food supply, and access to that supply for the growing urban poor in future decades, within the constraints of structural adjustment programmes which force controls on government spending for welfare and health. The World Bank defines food security as the provision to all people of 'enough food for an active, healthy life' (1986). The food security of urban populations may be affected by inadequate supplies of food, insufficient purchasing power to access that supply, or inefficient use of limited resources through choice or preparation of food and a background of ill-health.

After an introduction to aspects of these issues and some programme options available, this chapter explores the social aspects of urban populations, which have implications for food planning and for support to the economic activities of the urban poor through the informal sector.

## FOOD AND NUTRITION PROGRAMMES

### Food Supply

#### Commodity demand

Urban populations show a trend in the consumption of staples away from traditional, local roots or coarse grains (millet, sorghum and, to a lesser extent, maize) to wheat or rice. Although these grains are locally produced to some extent, the increased demand for them by the growing urban population often has to be met through increased imports (Delisle, 1989). Given the limited availability of foreign exchange, new approaches are needed to promote locally-produced foods, including research into the aspects of supply, processing, and convenience, which make these grains preferable in the urban setting, and into appropriate marketing strategies for local staples, which could be linked to price or income incentives.

In Sri Lanka, traditional sun-dried fruits and vegetables were used in local, rural areas but were not acceptable to the urban population. Products of an improved sun-drying method were acceptable to urban populations and had advantages over fresh, imported products, namely, longer shelf life, and more convenience and ease in preparation. The study identified minor improvements necessary in texture, taste, and flavour to ensure a successful small-scale industry of local, dried fruit and vegetables for an urban market (Delisle, 1989).

The contribution to total energy and nutrient intakes by staples decreases with urbanization, a trend mediated mostly by increased income. Therefore, food supply planning must also consider other sources of food, such as vegetables and fruits not necessarily produced by local farmers.

## Urban agriculture

Contrary to expectations, it has been demonstrated that urban agriculture has the potential to provide large amounts of food (Gutman, 1987) with surprisingly high yields (Wade, 1987). In the Far East, policies of urban or peri-urban food production have been pursued, although sometimes in an uncoordinated fashion (Yeung, 1987), and have been successful in providing the bulk of the demand from cities for commodities such as vegetables (Shanghai) and poultry (Singapore). This production for urban demand does not compete significantly with rural production and may provide opportunities for diversification into market gardening for peri-urban local farmers.

Governments need to revise their assumptions about the role of urban cultivation, and stop the harassment of urban cultivators while encouraging cultivation through grants and legal entitlements to land (Sanyal, 1985). Existing land use should be reviewed, and plans drawn up for temporary and multiple use of land, for example, along transport routes or around public institutions. Households could be encouraged to maximize space by using rooftops and balconies for gardening, and food production could be introduced in the process of upgrading low-income areas.

Water control is vital for urban agriculture which concerns the planning of drainage for flood control and the transport and distribution of water. Waste management could meet the demand for low-cost fertilizers by both home and market gardeners while, at the same time, addressing the problem of clearing refuse in cities, much of which is organic (Wade, 1987).

When the benefits of urban agriculture are compared with other urban food programmes (such as price subsidies, ration distribution, coupons), it is concluded that urban gardening cannot replace these. Those prepared to invest in the relatively long-term returns of agriculture are not the poorest or most recent migrants but lower-class workers and those of longer urban residence (Gutman, 1987). The advantage of urban agriculture is the promotion of self-reliance through using resources available in the community, minimizing the risk of benefits being diverted to other groups, and not damaging commercial farming.

Support to urban agriculture requires a bottom-up approach, with the use of extension workers as in a rural programme and a resource centre. It is expedient to launch the programme in those areas where there is already some self-help initiative, bolstering improvement and support to subsequent programmes through joint and evolving experience (Ninez, 1985).

## Access to Food

The commonest type of food and nutrition programmes are those that aim to improve nutrient intake through increased access to food. This may be achieved by direct feeding of, or food distribution to, identified beneficiaries; in effect, a means of income transfer to needy individuals and households. An alternative is to subsidize or control food prices which in theory allows the income of individuals and households greater purchasing power. The common use of nutritional status as the main indicator for monitoring these programmes points to an underlying assumption that food insecurity is defined by poor nutritional status, and that poor nutritional status arises primarily from inadequate food intake. This concept of food insecurity ignores other definitions such as poverty or vulnerability to food shortage with or without overt malnutrition (Maxwell, 1991).

### Direct feeding programmes

The direct approach provides supplementary food to pre-school children and pregnant and lactating women, usually through the health sector and through distribution of meals to school children, via the education or welfare sector.

Supplementary feeding programmes for children under five aim most commonly at the improvement of growth, prevention of growth failure, and/or reduction in the rates of malnutrition, and programmes are monitored through nutritional anthropometry. Such supplementary feeding programmes have had less impact on growth than expected, and a number of influences have been identified. Those most responsive to energy supplements are infants under three years and children with severe malnutrition (Kennedy and Knudsen, 1985; Freeman et al., 1977), particularly those classified as wasted by weight-for-height (<2SD). The growth response will depend also on the disease burden. Urban children from healthy environmental backgrounds in India had a more positive growth response to supplementary food than those from poor environmental backgrounds (Joshi and Rao, 1988).

The 'extra' food is not necessarily used as a supplement but may substitute home intakes or be shared with other family members. In six towns of Sao Paulo state, Brazil, home intakes of 50 per cent of preschool beneficiaries decreased, of which 65 per cent had inadequate total intakes (Mazzilli, 1987). The portion of energy that is incremental may not be used by the body for growth but for increased energy expenditure. After eight months of supplementation, urban pre-schoolers in Chile showed no change in nutritional status. However, fewer had sub-normal values of psychomotor development (Atalah *et al.*, 1989).

Similar issues arise with regard to school feeding programmes where nutritional status can be easily measured; improvements have been reported (Chen, 1989), but may not be as positive as expected, and other effects may be just as important but more difficult to assess. Urban children in Jamaica with a poor nutritional status, low attendance and achievement showed no effect on anthropometric indices with supplements but did show slight improvements in attendance and achievement (Powell *et al.*, 1983).

The use of supplementary food offers only a short-term solution but does not address the underlying causes of poor growth—and, indeed, may act to divert attention from these causes. Programmes in the distribution of supplementary food can be costly as they are often handled by trained health professionals. Such programmes are better understood as methods of effecting income-transfer rather than any direct, measurable health benefits. However, it is difficult to monitor the positive effects of income transfer on the health of a household and, moreover, supplementary food distribution may not be the most cost-effective way of making an income transfer.

## Community self-help schemes

There have been many small-scale initiatives, mainly undocumented and unsung, taken by communities themselves to use food more efficiently. Only two examples, already widely published, are given here to illustrate the potential of programmes for encouraging community action.

An innovative use of food aid in feeding programmes, involving community participation, has been made in urban areas of Peru. Food aid commodities are given to groups of women who make up a 'dining

room club'. They take it in turns to prepare morning and midday meals
in standard proportions which they then sell. Participants pay voluntar-
ily, according to their means, and the poorest families are allowed a free
meal. Each participant is entitled to a set number of servings per number
of household members. The funds collected go to buy foods supplement-
ing the basic commodities. The scheme has the advantage of reducing
the amount of time any household spends in food preparation, offering
opportunities for socializing and helping community members who are
not able to afford meals. The disadvantages are that individual tastes are
not catered to, and the control of food selection for the household and
method of preparation are removed from the person usually in charge of
this work (Katona-Apte, 1987).

Reviews indicate that the programme has nutritional benefits in that
participants are offered a wider variety of foods and eat more frequently
than non-participants, obtaining, on an average, 40 per cent of their daily
energy requirements (Martinez and Munoz, 1989). The monetary value
of the meals to a family is considerable as the cost is less than that of the
minimum food basket, even for those paying for the meal. The practice
of eating pre-prepared food does not affect usual eating patterns since
both participants and non-participants purchase a substantial amount of
the household's total food from outside sources. At the same time, the
provision of meals encourages adult males to eat at home—a factor considered to have a beneficial effect on family stability (Katona-Apte,
1987). Further, the programme is found to help families through periods
of economic crisis when food prices fluctuate, as meals can be bought at
standard rates (Saenz et al., 1989). Finally, the control of the programme
by women enhances their sense of value within the community.

In Karachi, Pakistan, on the Orangi Pilot project, community organization for construction and administration had been developed for a
sanitation programme. Building on this success, health and nutrition
education was started through women's groups. One of the important
spin-offs of the regular coming together of women was that they themselves identified common problems and organized food buying in bulk
at cheaper, wholesale prices.

## Indirect programmes of price control and food subsidy

Government policy has addressed the problem of inadequate access to
food for the urban poor sectors of the population through price controls
or food subsidies whereby certain basic commodities are sold at prices
lower than the true free market value. This can contribute substantially

to the income of poor consumers. Subsidized food ration schemes have been estimated to contribute 16 per cent in Sri Lanka, 13 per cent in Egypt, and 15–25 per cent in Bangladesh to incomes of the urban poor. Food consumption is estimated to have increased by 15–18 per cent in Kerala, India, and urban areas of Bangladesh (Pinstrup-Andersen, 1989). However, food subsidies should be seen only as compensatory short-term solutions rather than tools to achieve long-term goals.

Price control operates essentially as an income transfer from agricultural producers to the consumers, most of whom are urban. Such policies operate where producers are obliged to sell a given percentage of their crop to the government at a fixed price, or where producers themselves trade the crop but the market price is set at a legal maximum. Constraints on moving foodstuffs from one area to another may also be enforced to control black-marketeering in goods. The disincentive effects of such price controls on long-term agricultural production and development are now recognized as a cost that countries can no longer afford.

The alternative is to subsidize the sale of certain foodstuffs. This requires that government either buys from the producer at market price and sells at a lower price, or fixes the market price and compensates the farmer for the difference from the real market value. The effect of this is to depress prices on the market for the portion of the harvest sold independent of government purchase. Thus, unless subsidized food is sold through limited outlets, or farmers are compensated to the full extent of their crop—not just the part the government purchases—food subsidies again create cheaper food for the consumer supported by the producer. Subsidies also present a major drain on governments' budgets and thus need to be designed in the most cost-effective manner possible. Subsidies and price controls together are frequently used by governments in combination (Pemberton and Harris, 1988).

Programmes of structural adjustment have required major reductions in price controls and food subsidies, both because of the disincentives for agricultural producers and because of the huge costs to government. Such cuts have deleterious effects on access to food of those dependent on purchase of food, that is, the urban population, particularly the poor, as well as the poorest rural populations who are usually the landless labourers (Reutlinger, 1988). It has been argued that it is possible to design programmes that assist the poor consumer, mainly urban, without depressing prices of agricultural produce and with limited costs to government (Pinstrup-Andersen, 1989).

Food subsidies can be either untargeted or targeted to poor consumers through the choice of commodities subsidized and through the use of coupons, vouchers or stamps distributed according to a means test or through direct feeding to specific individual household members. Subsidies are almost always more cost-effective when targeted in some way, as long as the administrative costs of targeting do not outweigh the advantages (Kennedy and Alderman, 1989). It must be remembered that if a subsidy is too rigidly targeted to the poor, its political irrelevance is likely to threaten its continuation. In Colombia, a highly targeted, very cost-effective programme was terminated after four years as it was not politically important for the new government (Pinstrup-Andersen, 1989). The best option would appear to be the identification of a few basic staples which are predominantly used by the poor, but which can be subsidized for all, with or without further targeting by some means test for income or some other proxy indicator. (See also Chapter 7.)

## Direct or indirect nutrition programmes

Very few studies have made comparison of different types of programmes for their relative effects. Brazil has had a wide range of different 'experiments' and an evaluation has been made, retrospectively, of the effects of various programme types on nutritional status. Two programmes of direct supplementary feeding and two of food subsidy were compared, and a number of common assumptions questioned. The analysis supported the assumption that malnutrition is, above all, a consequence of poverty and, therefore, cannot be prevented or corrected without an economic transfer, but it was not evident that the price of food is the critical factor. There was also no evidence to show that poverty guarantees long-term participation in a programme; that a subsidy is cheaper to administer than direct feeding; that a subsidy is automatically transformed into a real benefit for the client or that the beneficiaries of a subsidy reach a final nutritional status as good as or better than that of participants in a direct feeding programme. The conclusion was that the economic diagnosis of malnutrition justifies direct intervention just as much as indirect subsidies. It was also stressed that the economic diagnosis is incomplete. The educational and medical components that often accompany direct feeding are crucial for improved nutritional status, particularly in infants under one year of age (Musgrove, 1990).

## Choice of Food

### Recent migrants

It has often been proposed that the move from rural to urban residence causes a decline in nutritional status as the family changes its dietary habits to the urban mode. The description of diet changes in Quito, Ecuador (Wichter *et al.,* 1988) includes a mixture, some of which a dietician would consider beneficial and some not, but it does not confirm a clear trend to a poorer diet. The case for nutritional stress during the transition period would be supported by evidence that nutritional status improves with length of residence. In Manaus, Brazil, length of residence was positively associated with family income, as was family income with adequate intake of energy and vitamin A. This implies a possible relationship of residency operating through increasing income, although length of residence itself was not significantly associated with nutritional adequacy (Amorozo and Shrimpton, 1984). On the other hand, a study of health factors in a slum in Rio de Janeiro, Brazil, found no association of a wide range of health indicators, including nutritional status, with length of residence (Reichenheim, 1988).

The proposition rests on the assumption that migrants arrive in the city as isolates. However, many urban communities retain links with their rural origins and kin if the rural home is relatively near (Logan, 1981; Kemper, 1981). Urban migrants may still have rural assets, will visit the rural home for festivals, often returning to the city loaded with foodstuffs (Kemper, 1981), and send children to the rural community for holidays and festivals. Likewise, rural population make use of their urban contacts for visits to the city, to send their children to better schools (or at least more accessible ones), and for assistance if someone is moving permanently to the city (Bossen, 1981). Therefore, although urban–rural migration undoubtedly involves stress through acculturation, most migrants do have some initial social contacts for support.

### Advertising

Urban populations are exposed far more to advertising than rural populations. The influence of advertising on food behaviour, the routes by which its influence operates, and the extent to which advertising is essentially operating as nutrition education (or mis-education), all need further study as little has been done beyond the baby milk industry. Advertising may work against sound nutrition practices by promoting unnecessary foods and by providing misleading information, particularly the suggestion that advertised foods are superior to other foods (Musaiger, 1983). Although the effects of advertising may be similar in developed and underdeveloped countries, the outcome is more serious in underdeveloped countries as misuse of foods aggravates the effects of poverty and ill-health. Further, there is less regulation of advertising in underdeveloped than developed countries (Musaiger, 1983). It is clear that advertising and other activities of the baby milk industry have an effect on both breast-feeding duration by mothers (Greiner and Latham, 1982) and, rather more insidiously, on attitudes of health professionals towards breast-feeding (Griffin *et al.*, 1984). Jelliffe (1972) coined the phrase 'commerciogenic malnutrition' to describe the outcome of the promotion of infant foods in areas where their use is seen as unsuitable.

Over the last twenty years, concern has moved from protein deficiency to energy insufficiency, but substantial investment has been made in developing protein-rich vegetable products which are still being promoted, although the claims are no longer valid and the costs can be 20–40 times as much as for adequate home-produced mixtures (Popkin and Latham, 1973). The promotion of protein-rich foods containing soya beans under USAID sponsorship, and the need to find export markets for USA soya bean harvests, is only one example of the importance of commercial interests (Pellet, 1976). Housewives of all socio-economic classes in Manama City, Bahrain, were found to respond to new advertisements for three products during the study period. Although the tendency to believe the claims of the promotion was highest amongst the poorest socio-economic groups, those not believing the claims also started purchasing the product—a feature that highlights the subtle nature of advertising (Musaiger, 1983).

In the Third World, there has been little study of consumer activities for programmes for facilitating consumer organization or techniques for consumer education. However, there is certainly great potential for consumer action in respect of food quality, particularly concerning safety and nutrient value of the food. Governments have not given sufficient priority to consumer education and organization in programmes of food security despite the potential contribution. The one area where consumer associations have been established, and have been successful, is in the monitoring of the marketing code for breast milk substitutes. This has shown the potential for consumer education and action to offset the interests of large transnational corporations (Delisle, 1989).

## Health Aspects

The interaction of nutritional status and infection has been frequently studied, and many thorough reviews exist (Tomkins and Watson, 1989). The major issues for the poor remain access to clean water, disposal of human waste and garbage, and drainage and housing quality (Satterthwaite, 1990). A few additional issues specific to the urban context are examined here.

### Industrial pollution

A specific concern of urban nutrition is how nutritional status interacts with exposure to environmental pollutants and industrial toxicants. A review of the literature of industrial toxicants and nutritional status indicates that poor status in any of a number of nutrients can increase the susceptibility to toxicity of substances (Atkinson, 1990). Recent work in Calcutta found that even where poor nutritional status may apparently lessen toxicity initially, the response is bi-phasic and, in the longer-term, is also associated with increased susceptibility. The Soviet Union used to explicitly incorporate a concern for nutritional status into occupational health services by providing workers with food high in those nutrients indicated by research to be protective (Sutphen, 1985). In Third World countries, many industrial enterprises are poorly controlled or are informal cottage industries, based in the home which can result in the local environment becoming badly contaminated (Barten, 1990). Risks from exposure thus concern all the local populations, not only those directly exposed through work. Occupational health services, including preventive nutrition advice, can be offered through community primary health services (Jayaratnam, 1989).

Child labour is common in cities where opportunities abound for exploitation of children. Health distress occurs overtly where children are 'asked or forced to do jobs known to be hazardous or unsafe for adults' (WHO, 1987). Covert exploitation is possible where children are 'asked or forced to do jobs that are generally considered to be safe for adults, but which are not necessarily safe for children because they are still in the period of growth and development' (WHO, 1987). Studies in pharmacology have indicated the necessity of adjustments of medication dosage by weight. There have been very few real-life studies of toxicant dose response in humans of any age, and although studies have been made on growing animals, these have not been translated into estimates of safe exposure levels, as most research has been carried out in the West in order to set exposure limits for adult workers (WHO, 1987). The metabolism of many toxicants is similar to that of drugs, so the same adjustments for safe doses are very probably necessary. In informal, small-scale industrial enterprises, child workers are likely to be in particular danger of toxicity. The interaction with poor nutritional status can only serve to exacerbate this further.

Another area of concern is the exposure to toxicants of pregnant and lactating women and the extent to which toxicants either affect the foetus or contaminate the mother's milk. The potential teratological effects of many toxicants have been studied in western countries, but there are no data on the interactions with nutritional status. Some studies have been made on the expression of pesticides, particularly of DDT, through breast milk, but the area is under-researched and, again, the interaction with poor nutritional status remains unexplored. (See also Chapter 1.)

## Food contamination

Food standards and their effective implementation for commercial foods will be of greater value to urban consumers than rural producers. Where recommendations or standards have been adopted, there is often not sufficient policing of products, and court cases can take a long time. The importance of food exports for the economy means that the majority of resources for routine sampling will be channelled into the export trade (Hobbs and Roberts, 1987). The major problems in food hygiene for tropical countries are caused by high temperatures, high humidity, lack of refrigeration, impure water, poor sanitation, and profusion of intestinal pathogens and parasites.

A comparison of campylobacter excreter rates in urban and rural Liberian children (6–60 months of age) revealed a higher urban excreter rate (Mølbak et al., 1988). The inverse relationship with water quality led to a further study which indicated that the higher urban excreter rates were due not to the contamination of water but to contamination of food. Urban families cooked and stored food more often, and stored food longer on average, than did rural families. The microbiological quality of urban stored food was particularly poor (Mølbak et al., 1989). Urban households prepared food only once a day and stored it longer because charcoal was expensive and also because mothers work long distances away from the home.

The use of street foods has been viewed as undesirable by governments as they are seen as costly and of low nutritional value. At the same time, there is a tendency to regard modern commercial food products as better than traditional ones in respect of nutritional value. The idea that street foods present a health hazard has been used widely by governments to denigrate street food and remove traders from the streets. Again, commercial preparations are promoted as superior in terms of hygiene. A four-city study of street foods belies the notions both of street foods being costlier and less nutritious and of commercial products having better nutritional quality. The study concludes that most street foods are probably safe if eaten soon after purchase. The safety of street foods needs to be assessed relative to other food sources. Conditions in many poor urban homes are little different from those on the streets, and neither vendors nor buyers will perceive any problems with street food hygiene (Tinker, 1987; Tinker and Fruge, 1982; Cohen, 1985).

## Child care

The relationship between use of commercial products and poor health and nutritional status is not straightforward but is mediated by other factors such as environment and income, (Zeitlin *et al.*, 1978; Khan and Gupta, 1977). In Guatemala, the children of working mothers in the better-paid formal and informal categories were breast-fed for a shorter time than the offspring of mothers in domestic work or in non-paid work, yet the former category of children had a better nutritional status. The authors explicitly relate this to increased income enabling mothers to afford the high density baby food INCAPARINA (Engle and Pedersen, 1989).

The question whether programmes promoting breast-feeding are realistic for all women in urban settings must be addressed. Many studies have indicated that the urban trend away from breast-feeding results predominantly from mothers going to work away from the home and thus being unable to continue breast-feeding (Anyanwu and Enwonwu, 1985; Ransome *et al.*, 1989). In these cases, promotion of breast-feeding may serve only to induce guilt in mothers and does not address their immediate need for a cheap, safe alternative.

A number of studies have examined whether the costs to child health from early cessation of breast-feeding are counteracted by the benefits of the extra income earned by the mother for the household, and the results are inconclusive overall. Studies of children of working mothers have revealed lower nutritional status (Powell and Grantham-MacGregor, 1985; Choudhary *et al.*, 1986; Popkin, 1980), no difference (Tucker and Sanjur, 1988) and better nutritional status (Tripp, 1981).

However, the model of a trade-off between the positive effects of increased income and the negative effects of decreased maternal child-care time is rather simple and overlooks a number of confounding factors. First, many women who opt for work outside the home are from poorer households than those women who do not, and therefore the variable of total income must be controlled in comparative analyses (Bennett, 1988; Engle and Pedersen, 1989). Secondly, the working conditions can vary greatly between different occupations and can have different effects on the children. Thirdly, the quality of alternative child care affects the outcome; family members make more responsible child supervisors than other people (Choudhary *et al.*, 1986; Tucker and Sanjur, 1988), and mothers working full-time organize more reliable care than those working sporadically or part-time (Wray and Aguirre, 1969). Lastly, maternal work will have different effects on different age groups.

The continued and increasing participation of women in the paid labour market requires a number of measures to enhance child care. Accordance with minimum wage legislation is often not applied to women, even in the formal sector, and differential wages may even be formally promoted on the basis that women provide merely a household's supplementary income (Barroso, 1989). The provision of good child-care facilities may have a major impact on child health. Brazil has legislated that all formal employers should provide creche facilities, but the impact of this kind of legislation has received little attention. The promotion of breast-feeding should continue, together with control of the promotion of substitute feeds. However, women working away from home will not be able to breast-feed, and substitutes that are easy to prepare, safe, cheap, and available in the local shops should be developed. In Benin, a local weaning mix was developed with UNICEF assistance and successfully marketed, partly through street food vendors (Delisle, 1989).

Many factors determining poor food security and a number of inter-related issues need to be considered by planners of programmes aimed at promoting food security. However, most of these factors are underpinned by poverty. The next section deals with the role of the household in the improvement of food security and the potential of the informal sector in securing the economic development of poor populations.

## SOCIAL ASPECTS OF PLANNING URBAN FOOD SECURITY

### Households

Food security at sub-national level is usually addressed by planners at the level of the household. Therefore, it is necessary to explore whether, and to what extent, the household is a meaningful economic unit in the urban context and to clarify the definition of household.

What constitutes a household has produced much debate. Most surveys focus on groups that share residence, domestic functions, kinship, or some combination of these features (Bender, 1967). Chant (1989) has developed a typology of urban households which outlines seven kinds, only five of which are based on kin. Both modernization and dependency theories predict a trend, with urbanization, from rural-extended households to urban-nuclear households, but this is not well supported. However, urbanization does seem to be associated with an increase in female-headed households in many parts of the world (Chant, 1989). Households can also be defined by long-term rather than current activities. Groups of individuals, usually with some kin relationship, may be jointly involved in long-term investment and petty capital formation outside the market sphere. In this definition of household, co-residence is de-emphasized as sharing a common residence is neither necessary nor by itself sufficient for membership (Bossen, 1981).

The implication in many definitions of household, and the use of the household as the unit for planning, is that the individual participates in the household strategies because it is largely to the advantage of the individual to do so in the short term or the long term. This is the argument of the joint utility function developed in the New Household Economics, which argues that the household acts to promote the common good of all its members (Piwoz and Viteri, 1985; Senauer, 1990). This position has been challenged by studies of household behaviour, showing that poverty does not affect all members of a household equally. There is a limited number of studies (none on an urban population) indicating that some household members are discriminated against within the household's allocation of scarce resources such as food (Piwoz and Viteri, 1985; Wheeler, 1988). Typically, inter-household allocation of food has been found to discriminate against young children and against females in certain circumstances and cultures.

Explanations for discrimination against women have concentrated on the social structure of cultures based on patriarchal systems. The comparison of North India, where marked sex differences are found in IMR, life expectancy, and nutritional status, with South India where these are not evident, has focused on the different role and status of women in the north and the south. Functional arguments have been offered that feeding the main breadwinner, usually the man, is a rational long-term strategy for a household. Underfeeding of young children has been explained as arising from misperceptions of energy needs. It has been suggested that children are fed as if their energy needs related to their size—whether weight, height, or surface area or some combination—without adequate understanding of the relationship between size and requirement (Wheeler, 1988). Most nutrition education programmes simply attribute the reason to ignorance, but studies on intra-household allocations, whether adopting functional or structural explanations, all suggest that the underlying causes are both more complex and more difficult to address than through the simple delivering of information.

In order to curtail discriminatory feeding, the bases of decision-making within the household have to be understood (Piwoz and Viteri, 1985). The power base of each household member within the household describes the relationships between family members, their relative bargaining power, and the influence of each in determining the use of household resources. The power base may reflect social status, which has traditionally been determined by the family structure, or economic importance to the household, determined by occupation or income. Within the urban household, the factors affecting the power base may be different from those found in the rural setting, and there is thus a need for urban studies.

Another aspect of individual interests, compared with those of the household, is the extent of food consumption outside the household. In Indonesia and the Philippines, urban households spent, on average, 25 per cent of their food budget on street foods (Tinker, 1987). Certain members of a household may get a substantial contribution of their daily energy intake outside the shared household resources, mostly from street vendors. Males in Hyderabad consumed up to 600 kcal per day away from the home. Urban secondary school children in Port-au-Prince, Haiti, acquired 25 per cent of their energy intake from street foods (Webb and Hyatt, 1988). This raises questions about the extent to which household members participate in the household through sharing of resources, and the extent to which they act as individuals. The use of either the individual or the household as the primary consumption unit is limiting in analyses of mechanisms of survival. Bossen (1981) promotes the idea that the individual is both part of an own egocentric reciprocity network and also a participant in household strategies. It is recognized that there is uncertainty in current literature as to when it is appropriate to focus on the economic behaviour of individuals, households, or networks (Bossen, 1981; Norris, 1988).

## Individuals

In addition to those operating partly in a household and partly as individuals, there are groups that merit special attention as not fitting into the standard conceptions of social organization.

The most evident social group, which falls completely outside of the usual family-residence definitions of household as the primary consumption unit, is children who do not belong to a family any more for various reasons. There is a certain amount of literature on the social life of street children (Agnelli, 1986; Aptekar, 1989; Ennew, 1986; Taçon, 1984), together with publications on numbers, working conditions, and so forth of child labourers in general (Challis and Elliman, 1979). Child labour is often a vital ingredient of a household's economy in the Third World. In urban populations, some children not only work from an early age but also leave their families, or are abandoned by them, and live by themselves or in gangs with other children. These are the true street children in the sense of street dwellers. In addition, many others work on the streets and interact with those who do not have families, sharing the same sources of food.

Child workers are often organized by adults into gangs and taken care of by the adults. In Seoul, Korea, boys are recruited as shoe-shiners through middle-men as they arrive in the city by train or bus. Shoe-shining is seen as preferable to other possible jobs such as working in cafes, as it is better paid, although the 'shoe-shine' gang is looked down upon by the rest of Korean society. The shoe-shine team is fed and housed by the territory boss, and works, eats, and lives together with limited scope for making contacts outside the team group. The shoe-shine organization draws upon the traditional Korean kinship system for the fundamental institutional framework. The direction of authority and respect follows age lines from father to son, and elder brother to younger brother. The territory boss is called 'father', and the supervisor of the team is called 'elder brother' (Kang and Kang, 1978). In this case, the gang with the supervisor and territory boss, operates rather like a household, although each member also has individual resources from earned income.

A study has recently been made on street children in Indonesia, and preliminary analyses have found that their nutritional status is nearly as good as that of children of high-income families and far better than children from low-income households. When life conditions become unbearable, children take the initiative if they have the chance, drop out of their family life, and demonstrate that they can live much better. This represents an explicit expression that the household does not always work in favour of all members and, under certain circumstances, children can survive better by acting as individuals or in groups with other children.

## Networks and Coping Strategies

Programmes to enhance urban food security may build on actions or strategies already adopted by individuals or households to generate income, with the aim of making these more effective. There is an increasing body of literature recording a range of coping strategies, especially those organized through the household.

The informal sector is used by the poor as a means to generate income for services rendered. It is noted that households with lower incomes are seen to engage in more activities, presumably trying to maximize the income-earning potential (Norris, 1988). Women are particularly active in this respect as they can draw upon home-making skills and extend them as a service. Thus, women may take in washing, sewing, set up a kindergarten, or work as maids and cleaners. Of particular interest for nutrition is the preparation and selling of pre-prepared food whether from the front doorway, on the streets, or through small cafes (Tinker and Fruge, 1982; Cohen, 1985; Tinker, 1987). Work as dance hall partners, bar girls, and prostitutes is common among single women heading households (Logan, 1981). Female household heads are engaged in the highest number of different income-earning activities and are the most impoverished. The better-off are more often engaged in formal market activities and tend to have only one income-earning activity.

Pooling incomes of a number of earners who share residence or food preparation can help cut costs. The commonest examples are where parents or other kin live with the family of the household head. Efficiency is maximized through using all available space, minimizing food waste, and developing ways to wash dishes, clothes, and people with minimum water. Objects are recycled for re-use. The recycling process itself provides income-earning opportunities through activities such as sewing (Logan, 1981). Some subsistence activities, such as raising small animals and small-scale urban agriculture, may be undertaken, as discussed earlier.

Some areas have established migrant associations which raise funds for local community projects. A similar form of redistribution of resources in the community operates through local forms of rotating credit.

These are largely run by women, and members contribute according to their means. Each week, one member receives the total sum contributed. This acts as a form of saving and capital accumulation (Kemper, 1981). Households have an important role as agents of capital accumulation in which certain kinds of income are withheld from current flows of goods and services and are instead turned into non-dispensable forms, such as housing, furniture, and appliances (Bossen, 1981). This investment in permanent goods represents an investment in long-term security, as these can be sold if times are hard in addition to improving current living standards.

There is a range of reciprocal exchange relations, used within the community, where services are exchanged and both parties gain in time saved. For example, one woman looks after the children while the other does the shopping for both. Reciprocal relationships may also be established between neighbours and work companions. In many societies, there are patron–client relationships where patrons can be called upon for assistance by their relatively impoverished clients. Examples of such a relationship include that of more fortunate kin assisting poor relatives, or the more formal compradrazgo system of Latin America (Norris, 1988).

Women are the major force in networks and coping strategies, as they run the local credit schemes, maintain the relationships of reciprocity, and are those most likely to be engaged in the greatest number of activities in the informal sector (Kemper, 1981). The importance of women's role in coping activities is particularly stressed as, in the past, it has often been overlooked.

These strategies can, however, achieve only so much, and coping by cost-cutting can prove deleterious to health and nutrition. Health care can be expensive and, if costs are cut in health expenditure, the adaptation may mean not seeking health care at all. Decreased expenditure on food is likely to mean substituting cheaper food items for those most preferred or consuming less of those preferred. Although there is no necessary relationship between the price of a food commodity and its nutrient content, substitution may lead to a more monotonous diet, which is more likely to be associated with a nutrient imbalance (Logan, 1981).

Women as income-earners are often at a special disadvantage, even in those countries where there are no obvious religious or moral constraints on women participating openly in the market. In formal employment, women often earn less for the same work, have access only to lower-paid jobs, and show little increment in income with experience (Barroso, 1989). In markets, women tend to be engaged in the retail of fruit, vegetables, and prepared foods and, although these are the bulk of items purchased from the market, they have the lowest profit margins and thus provide meagre incomes. In addition, men tend to have greater mobility to travel directly to the food production sites and can purchase goods directly from the producers at lower prices. Many male traders may also bring into the business income from other sources of employment. Although marketing is an occupation that women can combine relatively easily with domestic roles, the demands of their domestic work puts them at a structural disadvantage as traders relative to men (Babb, 1990).

## Informal Sector Development

The resourcefulness of the poor in generating income through informal employment and market activities has prompted debate on the extent to which the informal sector can be developed, not only to buffer the effects of periods of economic crisis for the poor but also to promote economic growth, productivity of the city, and absorption of surplus labour. The Zambian government stated, as early as in 1979, that it would rely heavily on the capacity of the informal sector to absorb the bulk of the labour force (Hansen, 1980). The vital issue in this debate is the relationship between the formal and informal sectors of the economy. Within the debate, two main positions on this relationship have emerged.

The relationship has been seen as a benign one, in which either goods and services were exchanged between the two sectors (Hart, 1973) or the informal sector was marginalized and autonomous (ILO, 1972). This benign model suggests that the informal sector has the capacity to generate, from within, surplus which is reinvested into the sector (Cornia, 1987). Policies can be developed to support the informal sector, increase its income-generating capacity, and enhance the surplus production.

The opposing model views the relationship of the informal to the formal sector as dependent and subordinate and that surplus generated in the informal sector is not retained or reinvested into the sector, and thus the accumulation of capital for launching a process of economic growth is not possible (Moser, 1978). The elasticity of the sector to absorb ever more labour during economic recession is also therefore limited (Tokman, 1978; Streefland, 1977).

The evidence suggests that there is no one answer, and the mistake is in viewing the informal sector itself as a homogeneous set of activities.

Relationships to the formal sector may be broadly categorized into three groups (Cornia, 1987). The growth potential of activities of small-scale contracting from the formal sector is obviously totally dependent on the growth of the formal sector. Activities of small-scale manufacturing provide goods for low- and middle-income consumers earning income from both formal and informal sources. Demand for such goods will be affected by competition with the formal sector. The informal sector has advantages in lower production costs, ability to acquire small markets, and convenience of location for certain goods. The relationship of this group of activities is thus only partly dependent on the growth of the formal economy in providing income for a segment of the consumers and its relative competitiveness. Lastly, activities of the retail trade, small-scale transport, and personal services are also provided to low- and middle-income consumers. There is little competition from the formal sector for these activities, so again the relationship only partly depends on the growth of the formal sector in providing income for a section of the consumers (Cornia, 1987).

The implication for planners is that a number of factors can and do operate to regulate and restrict the growth of the informal sector, that these vary in form and intensity by city, and that policies will have differential effects on different activities in the sector (Tokman, 1978).

It is striking that most of the key papers on the role of the informal sector as a source of income for the poor, and as a buffer against economic hardships, were carried out in the late seventies at the end of a period of economic expansion (Cornia, 1987). The World Bank (1991) has also highlighted the marked drop-off in all areas of social and economic urban research. The implications of this dramatically different macro-economic context for the apparent potential of the informal sector to generate economic growth and income for the urban poor are unknown.

There is obviously a need for scepticism in advocating informal sector support as the panacea for Third World urban problems. Although the economic activities of many of the urban poor would certainly benefit from not being subjected to harassment through government policy, it is still not clear in what ways assistance to small-scale, informal enterprises may best be extended without inadvertently producing negative effects.

## CONCLUDING OBSERVATIONS

Many of the studies in this chapter highlight the importance of not viewing the urban poor as a homogeneous population. There is a tendency to dichotomize populations into urban–rural, poor–rich, and informal–formal, whereas many studies have documented the variation in economic activities, income, social networks, and organization within communities identified as relatively deprived. A fuller picture of the mosaic of urban life is essential for development policy if realistic predictions are to be made of the likely impact of any policy on the nutrition of different social and economic groups.

Promoting urban food security requires coordinated planning across different sectors or ministries to address all the issues involved. The relevance of how and where people acquire their food, the social organization within which they do so, and the factors influencing their choices is often underestimated. Of importance for local level planning are the balance of individual action with household involvement, the influence of advertising on food choice, and the urban health issues of pollution, contamination, and exposure to toxicants. In respect of macro-economic planning, the crucial issues are how to avert the increasing demand for imported foodstuffs and to what extent the informal sector has the potential to provide employment, income, and economic growth for the city.

## REFERENCES

Agnelli, Susanna (1986). *Street Children: A Growing Urban Tragedy*, Weidenfeld and Nicolson, London.

Amorozo, Maria C. de Mello and Shrimpton, Roger (1984). The effect of income and length of urban residence on food patterns, food intake and nutrient adequacy in an Amazonian peri-urban slum population. *Ecol Food and Nutrition*, **16**, 307–23.

Anyanwu, Rosemary C. and Enwonwu, Cyril O. (1985). The impact of urbanization and socio-economic status on infant feeding practices in Lagos, Nigeria. *Food and Nutrition Bulletin*, **7**, 33–7.

Aptekar, Lewis (1989). Psychology of Colombian street children. *International Journal of Health Services*, **19**(2), 295–310.

Atalah, S. Eduardo *et al.* (1989). Evaluacion de un programa de alimentacion y estimulacion para prescolares de sectores de extrema pobreza. *Review of Child Nutrition*, **17**(supplement 1), 59–64.

Atkinson, Sarah J. (1990). *Diet and the Metabolism of Industrial Toxicants*. Centre for Human Nutrition, Department of Public Health and Policy, London School of Hygiene and Tropical Medicine.

Atkinson, Sarah J. (1992). *Food for the Cities: Urban Nutrition Policy in Developing*

*Countries*. Department of Public Health and Policy, Publication No. 5, London School of Hygiene and Tropical Medicine, London.

Babb, Florence E. (1990). Women's work: Engendering economic anthropology. *Urban Anthropology*, **19**(3), 277–302.

Baer, Roberta D. (1991). Inter- and Intra-household Income Allocation: Implications for Third World Food Policy. In: McMillan Della E. (ed), *Anthropology and Food Policy*, University of Georgia Press.

Barroso, Carmen *et al*. (1989). Impact of the crisis on the health of poor women: The case of Brazil. In: *UNICEF. The Invisible Adjustment*, UNICEF Regional Office for the Americas and the Caribbean.

Barten, Francoise J. M. (1990). Lead toxicity among children of urban slums situated in the vicinity of a battery factory in Nicaragua. MSc thesis CHDC, London School of Hygiene and Tropical Medicine.

Bender, D. R. (1967). A refinement of the concept of household: Families, co-residence and domestic functions. *American Anthropologist,* **69**, 493–503.

Bennett, Lynn (1988). The role of women in income production and intra-household allocation of resources as a determinant of child nutrition and health. *Food and Nutrition Bulletin*, **10**(3), 16–26.

Berg, Alan (1973). *The Nutrition Factor*. Brookings Institution, Washington, D.C.

Bossen, Laurel (1981). The household as economic agent. *Urban Anthropology*, **10**(3), 287–303.

Briscoe, John (1989). Adult health in Brazil. Unpublished Paper prepared for the World Bank.

Challis, James and Elliman, David, (1979). *Child Workers Today*. Quartermaine House.

Chant, Sylvia (1989). Gender and the urban household. In: Brydon, Lynne and Chant, Sylvia (eds), *Women in the Third World*. Edward Elgar.

Chen, S. T. (1989). Impact of a school milk programme on the nutritional status of school children. *Asia-Pacific Journal of Public Health*, **3**(1), 19–25.

Choudhary, M. *et al*. (1986). Nutritional status of children of working mothers. *Indian Pediatrics*, **23**, 267–70.

Cohen, Monique (1985). The influence of the street food trade on women and children. In: Jelliffe, Derrick, and Jelliffe, E. F. Patrice (eds). *Advances in International Maternal and Child Health*, Oxford University Press, Oxford.

Cornia, Giovanni A. (1987). Adjustment at the household level: Potentials and limitations of survival strategies. In: Cornia Giovanni A. *et al. Adjustment with a Human Face*. Oxford University Press, Oxford.

Delisle, Helene (1989). *Urban Food Consumption Patterns in Developing Countries*: *Some Issues and Challenges*, FAO, Rome.

Donahue, J. J. (1982). Facts and figures on urbanization in the developing world. *Ass Child*, **57/58**, 21–41.

Engle, Patrice L. and Pedersen, Mary E. (1989). Maternal work for earnings and children's nutritional status in urban Guatemala, *Ecol Food and Nutrition*, **22**(3), 211–23.

Ennew, Judith (1986). Children of the street. *New International*, 10–11 October.

Evenson, Robert E. (1981). Food policy and the new home economics. *Food Policy*, August, 180–93.

Freeman, Howard E. *et al.* (1980). Nutrition and cognitive development among rural Guatemalan children. *American Journal of Public He*alth, **70**, 1277–85.

Gilbert, Alan and Gugler, Josef (1981). *Cities, Poverty and Development: Urbanization in the Third World*, Oxford University Press, Oxford.

Greiner, Ted and Latham, Michael C. (1982). The influence of infant food advertising on infant feeding practices in St. Vincent. *International Journal of Health Services*, **12**(1), 53–75.

Griffin, Charles C. *et al.* (1984). Infant formula promotion and infant-feeding practices, Bicol Region, Philippines. *American Journal of Public Health*, **74**(9), 992–7.

Gross, Rainer and Monteiro, Carlos Augusto (1989). Urban nutrition in developing countries: Some lessons to learn. *Food and Nutrition Bulletin*, **11**(2), 14–20.

Gross, Rainer and Solomons, Noel (1985). Tropical urban nutrition. GTZ.

Gutman, Pablo (1987). Urban agriculture: The potential and limitations of an urban self-reliance strategy. *Food and Nutrition Bulletin*, **9**(2), 37–42.

Hansen, Karen T. (1980). The urban informal sector as a development issue: Poor women and work in Lusaka, Zambia. *Urban Anthropology*, **9**(2), 199–225.

Harpham, Trudy *et al.* (1988). *In the Shadow of the City*, Oxford University Press, Oxford.

Hart, Keith (1973). Informal income opportunities and urban employment in Ghana. *Journal of Modern African Studies*, **2**, 61–89.

Hobbs, Betty C. and Roberts, Diane (1987). *Food Poisoning and Food Hygiene*, (5th edn), Edward Arnold, London.

Hussain, Anwar M. and Lunven, Paul (1987). Urbanization and hunger in the cities. *Food and Nutrition Bulletin*, **9**(4), 50–61.

ILO (1972). *Employment, Incomes and Equality: A Strategy for Increasing Productive Employment in Kenya*, Geneva.

Jayaratnam, J. (1989). Special problems in developing countries. In: Waldron, H. A. (ed), *Occupational Health Practice*, (3rd edn), Butterworths.

Jelliffe, D. B. (1972). Commerciogenic malnutrition? *Nutrition Review*, **30**, 199–205.

Joshi, Smita and Rao, Shobha (1988). Assessing supplementary feeding programmes in selected balwadies. *European Journal of Clinical Nutrition*, **42**, 779–85.

Kang, Gay E. and Kang, Tai S. (1978). The Korean urban shoeshine gang: A minority community. *Urban Anthropology*, **7**(2), 171–83.

Katona-Apte, Judit (1987). Food aid as communal meals for the urban poor: The commedor programme in Peru. *Food and Nutrition Bulletin*, **9**(2), 45–8.

Kemper, Robert V. (1981). Obstacles and opportunities: Household economics of Tzintzuntzan migrants in Mexico City. *Urban Anthropology*, **10**(3), 211–29.

Kennedy, Eileen T. and Alderman, Harold H. (1989). Comparative analysis of the nutritional effectiveness of food subsidies and other food-related interventions: Conclusions. *Food and Nutrition Bulletin*, **11**(1), 74–6.

Kennedy, Eileen T. and Knudsen, Odin, (1985). A review of supplementary feeding programmes and recommendations on their design. In: Biswas, Margaret and Pinstrup-Andersen, Per (eds), *Nutrition and Development*, UNU/OUP, Oxford.

Khan, A. A. and Gupta, B. M. (1977). Social and economic factors in malnourished children around Lusaka, Zambia. *Tropical and Geographical Medicine*, **29**, 283–7.

Khanjanasthiti, Pensri and Wray, Joe D. (1974). Early protein–calorie malnutrition in slum areas of Bangkok municipality, 1970–1971. *Journal of the Medical Association of Thailand*, **57**(7), 357–66.

Logan, Kathleen (1981). Getting by with less: Economic strategies of lower income households in Guadalajara. *Urban Anthropology*, **10**(3), 231–46.

Martinez, Jacqueline and Munoz, Ana Maria (1989). Evaluacion nutricional de dietas de comedores familiares urbanos, Arequipa-Peru, *Review of Child Nutrition*, **17** suppl **1**, 25–30.

Maxwell, Simon (ed) (1991). *To Cure All Hunger: Food Policy and Food Security in Sudan*. IT Publications, London.

Mazzilli, Rosa Nilda (1987). A merenda no dia alimentar de criancas matriculadas em centros de educacao alimentacao do pre-escolar. *Rev Saude Pub*, **21**(4), 317–25.

Mølbak, Kare *et al.* (1988). High prevalence of campylobacter excretors among Liberian children related to environment conditions. *Epidemiology Information*, **100**, 227–37.

Mølbak, Kare *et al.* (1989). Bacterial contamination of stored water and stored food: A potential source of diarrhoeal disease in West Africa, *Epidemiology Information*, **102**, 309–16.

Moser, Caroline O. N. (1978). Informal sector or petty commodity production: Dualism or dependence in urban development, *World Development*, **6**(9/10), 1041–64.

Musaiger, Abdulrahman Obaid (1983). The impact of television food advertisements on dietary behaviour of Bahraini housewives. *Ecol Food Nutrition*, **13**, 109–14.

Musgrove, Philip (1990). Do nutrition programmes make a difference? The case of Brazil. *International Journal of Health Services*, **20**(4), 691–715.

Niñez, Vera (1985). Working at half potential: Constructive analysis of home garden programmes in the Lima slums with suggestions for an alternative approach. *Food and Nutrition Bulletin*, **7**(3), 6–14.

Norris, William P. (1988). Household survival in the face of poverty in Salvador, Brazil: Towards an integrated model of household activities. *Urban Anthropology*, **17**(4), 299–321.

Pellett, Peter L. (1976). Nutritional problems of the Arab world. *Ecol Food Nutrition*, **5**, 205–15.

Pemberton, Carlisle A. and Harris, Emeline L. (1988). Determining the beneficiaries of cheap-food policies in Trinidad and Tobago. *Food and Nutrition Bulletin*, **10**(4), 59–65.

Pinstrup-Andersen, Per. (1989). Food subsidies in developing countries. *Food and Nutrition Bulletin*, **11**(2), 74–8.

Piwoz, Ellen G, and Viteri, Fernando E. (1985). Studying health and nutrition behaviour by examining household decision-making, intra-household resource distribution, and the role of women in these processes. *Food and Nutrition Bulletin*, **7**(4), 1–31.

Popkin, Barry M. (1980). Time allocation of the mother and child and nutrition. *Ecol Food Nutrition*, **9**, 1–14.

Popkin, Barry M. and Bisgrove, Eilene Z. (1987). Urbanization and nutrition in low income countries. In: *Symposium on Nutritional Effects of Urbanization*, 13th Session of UN Co-ordinating Committee on Nutrition. PAHO, Washington, DC.

Popkin, B. M. and Latham, M. C. (1973). The limitations and dangers of commerciogenic nutritious foods, *American Journal of Clinical Nutrition*, **26**, 1015–23.

Powell, Christine A. and Grantham-McGregor, Sally (1985). The ecology of nutritional status and development in young children in Kingston, Jamaica, *American Journal of Clinical Nutrition*, **41**, 1322–31.

Powell, C. *et al.* (1983). An evaluation of giving the Jamaican school meal to a class of children. *Human Nutrition: Clinical Nutrition*, **37**(5), 381–8.

Pryer, Jane (1990). *Socio-Economic Aspects of Undernutrition and Ill-Health in an Urban Slum in Bangladesh*, Oxfam Health Unit, Oxford.

Ransome, O. J. *et al.* (1989). Factors influencing breast-feeding in an urban community. *South African Medical Journal*, **76**(8), 431–3.

Reichenheim, Michael Eduardo (1988). *Child Health in an Urban Context*. London School of Hygiene and Tropical Medicine and Institute of Child Health, PhD thesis, London.

Reutlinger, Shlomo (1988). Urban malnutrition and food interventions. *Food and Nutrition Bulletin*, **10**(1), 24–8.

Saenz, Nair Carrasco *et al.* (1989). Experiencia de apoyo y evaluacion nutricional a un comedor comunal en Lima metropolitana. *Rev Chil Nut*, **17** suppl 1, 55–8.

Sanyal, Bishwapriya (1985). Urban agriculture: Who cultivates and why? A case study of Lusaka, Zambia. *Food and Nutrition Bulletin*, **7**(3), 15–24.

Satterthwaite, David (1990). Urban and industrial environmental policy and management. In: Winpenny, J. T. (ed). *Development Research: The Environmental Challenge*, ODI, London.

Schurch, B. and Favre, A. M. (1985). *Urbanization and Nutrition in the Third World*. Nestle Foundation, Lausanne.

Senauer, Benjamin (1990). Household behaviour and nutrition in developing countries. *Food Policy*, October, 408–17.

Solomons, Noel and Gross, Rainer (1987). Urban nutrition in the tropics: A call for increased attention to metropolitan population in the developing world. *Food and Nutrition Bulletin*, **9**(2), 43–4.

Streefland, Pieter (1977). The absorptive capacity of the urban tertiary sector in Third World countries. *Development and Change*, **8**, 293–305.

Sutphen, E. I. (1985). Soviet prophylactic nutrition for workers in toxic chemical occupational environments, *American Journal of Child Nutrition*, **42**(4), 746–8.

Taçon, Peter (1984). Dignity in the streets, *UNICEF News*, **121**, 18–19.

Tinker, Irene (1987). Street foods. *Current Society*, **35**(3), 1–110.

Tinker, Irene and Fruge, Michelle (1982). The street food project. *Ass child*, **57/58**, 191–200.

Tokman, Victor E. (1978). An exploration into the nature of informal–formal relationships. *World Development*, **6**(9/10), 1065–75.

Tomkins, Andrew and Watson, Fiona (1989). *Malnutrition and Infection: A Review*. Clinical Nutrition Unit CHN, London School of Hygiene and Tropical Medicine, London.

Tripp, R. B. (1981). Farmers and traders: Some economic determinants of nutritional status in Northern Ghana. *Journal of Tropical Pediatrics*, **27**, 15–22.

Tucker, Katherine and Sanjur, Diva, (1988). Maternal employment and child nutrition in Panama. *Social Science and Medicine*, **26**(6), 605–12.

Viteri, Fernando E. (1987). Nutrition-related health consequences of urbanization. *Food and Nutrition Bulletin*, **9**(4), 33–49.

Wade, Isabel (1987). Community food production in cities of the developing nations, *Food and Nutrition Bulletin*, **9**(2), 29–36.

Webb, Ryland E. and Hyatt, Susan A. (1988). Haitian street foods and their nutritional contribution to dietary intake. *Ecol Food Nutrition*, **21**, 199–209.

Wheeler, Erica (1988). *Intra-Household Food Allocation: A Review of Evidence.* Occasional Paper No. 12 CHN, London School of Hygiene and Tropical Medicine, London.

WHO (1987). *Children at Work: Special Health Risks*, WHO, Technical Report Series, No. 756, Geneva.

Witcher, Bethann *et al.* (1988). Influence of rural–urban migration on adult women's food patterns and adequacy of their children's diet in Ecuador. *Ecol Food Nutrition*, **21**, 189–98.

World Bank (1986). *Poverty and Hunger: Issues and Options for Food Security.* World Bank, Washington, D.C.

World Bank (1991). *Urban Policy and Economic Development: An Agenda for the 1990s.* World Bank, Washington, DC.

Wray, J. D. and Aguirre, A. (1969). Protein–calorie malnutrition in Candelaria, Colombia. 1. Prevalence, social and demographic causal factors. *Journal of Tropical Pediatrics*, **15**, 76–98

Wray, Joe D. (1986). Child health interventions in urban slums: Are we neglecting the importance of nutrition? *HPP*, **1**(4), 299–308.

Yeung, Yue-Man. (1987). Examples of urban agriculture in Asia. *Food and Nutrition Bulletin*, **9**(2), 14–23.

Zeitlin, M. *et al.* (1978). Breast-feeding and nutritional status in depressed urban areas of Greater Manila, Philippines. *Ecol Food Nutrition*, **7**, 103–13.

# 4

# Nutrition and Ageing in Development

MARK L. WAHLQVIST, WIDJAJA LUKITO, AND
BRIDGET H-H. HSU-HAGE

## INTRODUCTION

By the year 2001, about 60 per cent of the human population aged 65
years and above will be those of the developing world (Andrews, 1986).
This indicates a 78 per cent net increase in the age group 65 years and
above in developing countries in the period 1980 to 2000. The experience of the developed world shows that the rapid increase in life
expectancy of elderly people generates a disproportionate increase in
medical expenses and health care costs (Ogawa, 1982). Given that we
are only seven years away from the year 2001, we anticipate as much, if
not greater, urgency in the consideration of health-related problems, particularly that of nutrition and ageing, besetting people 65 years and over,
in the developing world.

Nutrition plays an important role in the health status of a population.
Nutritional standard is a function of socio-cultural factors, food intake,
and intrinsic biology, with genetic and other environmental determinants. Biological processes, such as ageing, may also be a function of
nutritional status. A study of nutrition and ageing therefore needs to take
account of individual and population differences in socio-cultural factors
and biology.

We will consider nutrition–health relationships in the aged, and lessons from the Western Pacific, Meso-American, and IUNS (International
Union of Nutritional Sciences) studies of the elderly, before arriving at
general conclusions and implications for the future.

## NUTRITION–HEALTH RELATIONSHIPS IN THE AGED

### Derivation of the Relationships

Ageing is often accompanied by the occurrence of *illness, which may increase the risk of nutritional deficiency*. On the other hand, nutritional deficiency or excess may *contribute to the pathogenesis of a number of common diseases* of the elderly. Therefore, a description of the well-being and health status of the elderly has to take into account the nutritional status.

Nutritionally-related problems are often compounded by *diminished physiological reserve* in the elderly. Many studies have shown significant changes in different body functions while ageing. Some of the impaired functions are cardiorespiratory (Shephard, 1986), gastrointestinal (Duthie and Bennett, 1963; Webster, 1980), liver and renal (Thompson, 1963; Dontas *et al.*, 1972; Lindeman *et al.*, 1985), endocrine (Davidson, 1979; Friedman *et al.*, 1969; Riggs and Melton, 1986), and neurological (Sandman *et al.*, 1987; Bucht and Sandman, 1990)—and they may sometimes be nutritionally reversible. On the other hand, if 'nutritional reserve' is also limited (say, by reduced energy stores and nutrient stores in liver, muscle, and bone), then diminished physiological reserves of other kinds may be more critical. Thus, nutritional modulation by means of prevention and therapy represents one possible approach to the minimization of the occurrence of nutritionally-related health problems.

If we understand how to match food to biological need, and learn to identify common health problems and the nature of nutrition–health relationships while, at the same time, discerning the impact of non-nutritional factors on health, we will be in a better position to study and improve the health of the aged.

### Matching Food to Biological Need

It may not be unusual to assume that *food excess* amongst the elderly in developed countries and *food deficiency* in developing countries would characterize and separate the health problems in these settings (Table 4.1). However, although obesity is more common in developed than developing countries (WHO, 1990), with advancing years, there can be in both situations a decline in lean mass with a range of fat masses. The reduced lean mass puts both groups of elderly people at potentially similar risk from disorders related to it *per se*, for instance, immunodeficiency (Saltzman and Peterson, 1987). Indeed, it may be more help-

**Table 4.1** Putative role of nutrients in the pathogenesis of some diseases in the elderly

| Food intake patterns | Nutrient considerations | Disease | Relative prevalence Developed countries | Developing countries |
|---|---|---|---|---|
| High-energy density foods | Positive energy balance | Obesity | ++ | + |
| | | Hypertension | ++ | ++ |
| | | Non-insulin dependent Diabetes mellitus | ++ | + |
| Preference of salt and/or soysauce as flavour over herbs and spices | Excess sodium intake | Hypertension | + | + |
| | | Cerebrovascular accident | + | + |
| High plant-derived foods | High-fibre diets | Volvulus | + | + |
| Limited food supply | Protein–energy malnutrition | Immune deficiency | + | ++ |
| | | Anaemia/fatigue | + | ++ |
| | | Increased infection | + | +++ |
| Preference for animal-derived foods and/or fat | Low-fibre diets | Diverticulitis | ++ | + |
| | | Constipation | ++ | ++ |
| Limited variety or vegetarian diet | Folate and vitamin $B_{12}$ deficiency | Anaemia | + | ++ |
| | | Dementia | ++ | ++ |
| Limited dairy products and fish | Decreased calcium and vitamin D intake | Osteopenia and osteomalacia | ++ | ++ |
| Low meat and cereal intake | Zinc deficiency | Immune deficiency | ++ | ++ |
| | | Anorexia | ++ | ++ |
| | | Poor wound healing | + | ++ |
| Low meat and/or lack of combined intake of meat, fish, and green vegetables | Iron deficiency | Anaemia | + | +++ |
| Limited safe water supply | Hypoditisia | Dehydration | + | ++ |
| | | Orthostatic hypotension | + | ++ |
| | | Hypernatraemia | + | ++ |

+ low prevalence; ++ moderate prevalence; +++ high prevalence

References: Bjorntorp, 1990; Chandra, 1982; Davidson, 1979; Flint *et al.*, 1981; Herbert, 1962; Krishnan, 1974; Meydani *et al.*, 1990; Riggs *et al.*, 1986; Rolls, 1990.

**Table 4.2** Various food/body tissue deficit or excess in the elderly

|          | Food | | | Body tissue | | | |
|----------|--------|---------|-------|--------|------|-----|------|
|          | Energy | Quality | Water | Saline | Lean | Fat | Bone |
| Deficit  | +      | +       | +     | +      | +    | +   | +    |
| Excess   | +      | −       | ±     | +      | −    | +   | −    |

+ observed in the elderly
± rarely observed in the elderly
− never observed in the elderly

ful to refer to food deficit or food excess and lean mass and/or fat mass disorders in their own rights (Table 4.2).

Problems currently related to such classification are: (1) available definitions generally apply to younger adults, for example, nutrient density of food in mass or energy value, chronic energy undernutrition is BMI less than 18.5 kg/m$^{-2}$ (James *et al.*, 1988); and (2) no definitions exist or are only now being evaluated, for example, food variety score for nutritional counselling (Wahlqvist, 1989). Fortunately, food–health relationship studies, now in progress, will begin to solve these dilemmas.

Again, even 'nutritional quality' can be an inadequate descriptor if all that is nutritionally important in food is not considered. For example, dietary fibre intake varies greatly within and between the developed and developing worlds. Whereas the diet of certain developing countries may be regarded as low in dietary fibre, this may not be so for resistant starch, provided by rice and wheat noodles in an Oriental diet, where food is eaten after cooking (gelatinization of starch) and allowing it to cool somewhat (crystallization of starch). In this event, the function of dietary fibre attributable to its fermentation in the colon may be fulfilled as well, if not better, by resistant starch. But the accompaniments of dietary fibre and resistant starch may be quite different.

A cross-sectional study of Melbourne Chinese revealed that the intake of steamed rice did not alter with age. There were apparent increases in the intake of Chinese tea, Chinese cabbage, and beancurd while the consumption of beansprout decreased with age (Hage, 1992). Although it is likely that cohort effects may be operational, with age, food preference may be for foods with less 'roughage' (dietary fibre), but no less for resistant starch (Fig. 4.1). Thus, food intake may match some biological needs, but not all, and this may change with age and in accordance with food culture and socio-economic status.

The overall *food supply*, type of food production, food technology,

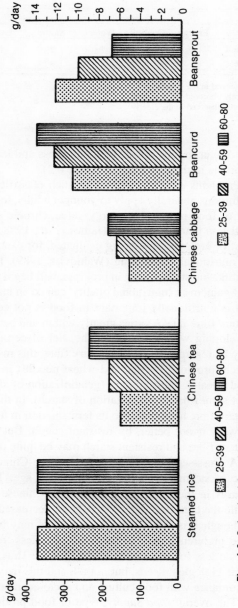

**Fig. 4.1** Selected food intakes in Melbourne Chinese (different age groups)

and food storage may peculiarly benefit or handicap elderly people at different stages of development. For example, elderly people may be vulnerable, with seasonal change or famine, in one developing country in a way that is transcended by the curing and salting of food in another developing society, or by the canning and freezing of food in an industrialized society. Opportunity to manage monetary matters, and therefore food resources, can also be critical. These relate to *food security* for the elderly (Arnauld *et al.*, 1990). Once life expectancy increases, *age-related diseases* also tend to increase. These health hazards can have their own impact on nutritional status. For example, the advent of diabetes mellitus, whose prevalence increases with advancing years, can alter nutritional needs, and require dietary modifications which may include restriction in accordance with attendant risk. Wasting diseases such as cardiac cachexia, or cerebrovascular disease with disability that impairs food preparation and the ability to eat, present unique sets of food needs. The *management of disease and disability* in the aged can also contribute its own set of nutritional problems. This is particularly evident in pharmacotherapy with adverse effects of drugs on appetite and taste, and nutrient absorption and handling (Roe, 1984).

International comparisons suggest that health problems in developing countries tend to follow those of developed countries in the course of industrialization (Gopalan, 1992). However, in transition, the problems can be mixed and complex, as evidenced by concomitant abdominal obesity and protein malnutrition or nutritional anaemia. An understanding of these nutritionally-related health problems in the aged in developed countries provides an opportunity to examine future trends in global health problems.

## Nature of the Relationship

### Nutritional dissimilarity and commonality

It is noteworthy that in developed, transitional, and developing countries, individuals survive to old age, witnessing different nutritional problems and disease patterns. There is therefore a challenge to ensure that, with ever-changing socio-cultural and socio-economic conditions, the fundamental characteristics of food culture, which confer well-being, health, and longevity, are identified and retained (Table 4.3). It is becoming apparent that peoples of all nations with different food cultures may have comparable life expectancy and morbidity rates (Powles, 1992). The challenge is to identify those food factors and patterns in common

**Table 4.3** Considerations in the retention of traditional practices, and intakes in developed and developing societies

| Developed society | | Developing society | |
|---|---|---|---|
| Favourable | Discouraged | Favourable | Discouraged |
| Live longer | Monoculture | Local food supply | Urbanization |
| Cultural assertive- | Rapid change of | Local food technol- | Advent of elec- |
| ness | food technology | ogy | tricity |
| | | Oral tradition | Media |
| | Food transport | Road in access | Education |
| | Supermarket | Respect for the el- | Migration |
| | | derly | |
| | Travel | | |
| | Restaurants | | |

between cultures that confer less morbidity and lower mortality (Wahlqvist *et al.*, 1993). To make this deduction requires an analysis of food intake in terms of overall mathematical descriptors of food patterns, category of food ingested, or the unifying value of a particular component of food, either nutrient or non-nutrient. For example, the extent of food variety may be an index of a favourable food pattern and culture. Fish intake may explain how the apparently disparate food cultures of Scandinavia, the Mediterranean, and Japan, all confer longevity (Briggs and Wahlqvist, 1988). The low intake of saturated fat may be a unifying nutrient indicator of biological advantage with respect to food culture. The class of compounds with weakly oestrogenic properties may be an example of non-nutrients which benefit people in later life and across food cultures (Wilcox *et al.*, 1990; Lee, 1992).

## Antecedents of being elderly and the nutrition–health relationship

*The present-day elderly* in the occident are peculiarly advantaged on the whole, having been provided with social welfare facilities beyond retirement, or the support of younger people, and not being subjected to the economic burden of a large aged population as they move through adulthood. The next generation of elderly in industrialized society may not be so fortunate, but rather may be more akin to the current generation in developing and transitional societies. In other words, industrialized societies may yet have something to learn from what is happening amongst the elderly in developing countries. At the same time, the transfer of food–health knowledge from grandparent (as many as all foregrandparents) to grandchild has never been as feasible as at present, because of the major gains in life expectancy. Thus, the future generation of elderly may be unusually enriched by such knowledge, depending on the respect accorded to elders.

*What constitutes 'life expectancy at birth'* is an artificial aggregate of the current experience of performance in different age brackets. Therefore, we may never witness exactly the same antecedents of being elderly as at present, for example, the experience of one or two great depressions and two major wars (if not more local ones). It is difficult to gauge the success of later life, in spite of, or because of, periods of privation in earlier life and, therefore, to assess how much present food–health relationships are operative because of these antecedents. Our presumption is that what operates now amongst survivors into later life can operate again. And this may be a range of eating behaviours or patterns for comparable health (Wahlqvist *et al.*, 1993).

*Urbanization* is one of the most urgent changes for young and old alike, with its implications for nutrition. The UN and WHO statistical data suggest that mortality is primarily influenced by socio-economic development measures such as urbanization, industrialization, and education, and secondarily by such public health measures as access to safe water, adequate nutrition, and health services (Rogers, 1989). Moreover, in less industrialized countries, urbanization could contribute to improvement in food habits (Dupin, 1974). However, urbanization may also create structural disruption and social disintegration which contribute to a disease-prone environment (Griffin, 1975). These processes may operate in part through dislocation of the food supply. For the rural elderly, especially elderly women, who may be left behind, the urbanization of youth in search of employment, and who otherwise may have supported them, may aggravate their nutrition problems. Nutritional problems of older women in rural homes may need more attention. Sometimes economic benefit to those left behind does accrue from the younger migrant or itinerant member of the family. Collections of letters home, in which cheques have been enclosed, bear testimony to this.

Major differences are emerging between the health patterns of urban and rural areas in the developing world. For example, the prevalence of high blood pressure in both men and women is at least four times as high in the urban as in the rural areas of Ghana (Pobee, 1980). Such phenomena are caused partly by the fact that urban societies tend to perceive the new diet, similar to that of other affluent communities, as a symbol of their newly-acquired status. Where the extended family still exists, new lifestyles and 'modern' diet may have an impact on the health of elderly people. However, presumptively, the rural elderly may be spared these changes more than their urban counterparts.

*Socio-economic development* in developing countries is followed by improved health care and better access to modern health technology, and these will promote the decline in mortality rate and increase in life expectancy. The dominant feature of this transition has been the progressive ageing of population. This *demographic transition* is clearly estimated by the population projection. For example, the total population of the countries of South-East Asia Region (SEAR), which stood at nearly 1053 million in 1980, is expected to increase to 1980 million by the year 2050; this represents a two-fold increase. During the same period, the number of the elderly (above 60 years of age) will increase from approximately five per cent to 11.5 per cent of the total population. In absolute terms, there will be a four-fold increase (173 million) in people older than 60 years of age in SEAR countries in the period 1980 to 2050 (Gopalan, 1992). On the other hand, during this time, the percentage of children under four years will decrease.

For developing countries, as in the developed world, the *costs of health care* for the elderly, at risk now—not only of nutritional problems previously expressed in their generational counterparts, when they were younger, but also of various chronic diseases—may be overwhelming. Experience in Japan has shown that the share of Gross National Product (GNP) required for the medical care of the elderly will rise from five per cent in 1986 to over six per cent in 2020, and the share of the national income to support this will climb from 6.3 to 8.7 per cent (Ogawa, 1982). These projections are alarming insofar as the maintenance of the health status and nutritional status of the elderly are concerned.

Even in developed countries, the elderly are vulnerable to undernutrition and specific nutrient deficiencies (Flint and Wahlqvist, 1981). In most cases, the elderly in developing countries will be more exposed to these nutritional problems. The dietaries in developing countries, for example in most Asian countries, are predominantly cereal-based, with relatively low concentrations of proteins, vitamins, and minerals. Thus, the risks of essential nutrient deficiency are extremely high. Nutrition education about nutrient-dense food and the value of food variety ought to minimize the occurrence of nutritionally-related health diseases in later life, but the food supply and its affordability in an urbanizing, mobile, and dislocated society may mitigate the effectiveness of such education. Family and social cohesion, along with de-emphasis on retirement and encouraging the continuation of even a partial livelihood through personal effort, may provide sufficient network and independence to affording a reasonably adequate diet.

## Work patterns and nutrition amongst the elderly

*Agriculture* is a major economic and social activity in developing countries. Various studies show a positive effect of nutritional intervention on agricultural production, especially for activities in which the poor, including the aged poor, are engaged. Among the sugarcane workers in Guatemala, productivity increased with improved nutrition. In Indonesia the productivity of workers who received iron supplements for two months rose to 15–25 per cent (World Development Report, 1990). A study in India showed a significant link between wages and weight-for-height among casual agricultural labourers (Khandker and Shahidur, 1989). Another study revealed that the effect was especially marked in the peak agricultural season, when more energy is required for harvesting (Ferro-Luzzi *et al.*, 1990).

Many studies show a close link between *retirement and poverty* in the aged. With longer life expectancy in women, the likelihood of poverty amongst elderly women is greater than for elderly men; over 50 per cent of aged women in the poverty bracket are widows (Kahne, 1981). Further, the period of retirement lengthens as the population ages (Leeds, 1981). These problems are accentuated by *inflation* which makes it more difficult to meet—even with a lifetime of saving—expenditure needs, including those for foods. In addition, the elderly may be less adaptable insofar as expenditure in relation to food choice is concerned. Poverty in old age may also be a function of low socio-economic status prior to retirement, depressed social status of the retired, or the relatively low level of state benefits (Walker, 1981). Whatever the cause, poverty affects food intake, nutritional status, and health.

## Non-nutritional Factors Affecting Nutritional Status and Health of the Aged

Various non-nutritional factors require special consideration in the aged. These may, on the one hand, affect food habits, food practices, and therefore intake in the elderly, and on the other hand affect nutritional needs. Of particular importance are: cultural factors which include food and health beliefs; social and psychological factors; economic factors; and physical activity and substance abuse.

## Cultural factors

Food habits are based in culture, and are more likely to be adhered to by the older members of the society. Again, traditional values are more widespread in developing than in industrialized countries, and within a population the oldest sector is the strongest basis of these values (Solomons, 1992). The extent to which grandchildren and great-grandchildren inherit the food beliefs and practices from their forebears will influence their ultimate nutritional status. In an extended family engaging in subsistence agriculture, the elderly often continue to work physically with favourable benefits for increased energy intake, with less obesity than might otherwise obtain, and with retention of lean mass (Wahlqvist and Kouris, 1990).

## Social and psychological factors

Research has demonstrated the close links between social and psychological factors and dietary intake in the elderly. Sub-groups of an elderly population in Adelaide, Australia, identified as being at a higher risk of poor dietary intake were: men living alone, low socio-economic status groups, and the socially isolated or physically inactive (Horwath, 1989). Some of these sub-groups will equate with those in developing countries (Table 4.4). Lifestyle, as measured in terms of participation in a variety of social and physical activities, was a good predictor of dietary intake, a varied lifestyle being associated with a varied diet. Prospective studies

**Table 4.4** Factors contributing to protein-energy malnutrition in the elderly

| | |
|---|---|
| Sociological factors | Socio-economic status |
| | Housing |
| | Residency |
| | Marital status/children |
| | Erroneous belief and food faddism |
| | Season |
| Psychological factors | Ethnic/cultural factors |
| | Cognitive functioning |
| | Sense of control and health-related behaviour |
| | Hypochondriasis and perceived intolerence |
| | Food preference |
| Physiological factors | Health |
| | Motor performance and mobility |
| | Senses |
| | Dental status |
| | Chronic disease |
| | Drugs |

showed that increased social activity and/or wider social network were associated with a lower mortality rate in the elderly (Olsen *et al.*, 1991; Silverstein and Bengtson, 1991). Much social activity revolves around food, which thereby assumes an important health-promoting function, aside from the provision of nutrients. Loss of spouse and bereavement also have significant effects on nutritional status and the immune system in the elderly (Davies, 1990; Chandra, 1990, 1990a).

In most developing countries, social and cultural patterns continue to protect the elderly from isolation in society. Self-care by older people themselves, and informal care by family and neighbours, can operate most effectively. WHO studies in the Western Pacific reveal that a large proportion of older persons have their needs met by their children or next of kin (Andrews, 1986). In each of these situations, food and nutrition is one of the vehicles for health benefit.

## Economic factors

As discussed earlier, poverty in developing countries affects the elderly and their food intake. It operates in various ways. Restricted income limits education and health services as determinants of health status. Poverty-induced rural–urban migration may deprive elderly people of immediate support from the younger generation, notwithstanding the potential for income generation from the remote family (Andrews, 1986). Dependence on those who are still productive signifies vulnerability, however. The aged, with a limited local food supply and reduced contact, are less able to pass on their food knowledge and skill.

It is possible that the effects of poverty could be limited if there were an adaptive response to limited energy intake. It does so, in relation to seasonal fluctuations in energy balance, where adult men and women are in negative energy balance during the hungry season and in positive balance during the post-harvest season. There appear to be biological-genetic, metabolic, and behavioural mechanisms for adaptation to low energy intakes (Ferro-Luzzi, 1990). These adaptive responses are directed towards energy conservation and eventually to the restoration of energy balance. Regrettably, there is little information on this adaptive response in the elderly.

## Physical activity

The role of physical activity in the maintenance of preferred nutritional status is crucial, and this is unlikely to be any more or less important in relation to development. This is principally because the decline in physical activity (Astrand, 1968), energy intake, and lean mass is more or less in parallel with advancing years (Smith *et al.*, 1988; Steen, 1988). However, it must be acknowledged that no good cross-sectional or longitudinal data on this matter exist for elderly people in developing countries. Not only should the maintenance of physical activity allow for a better body composition (more lean, less fat, more bone), but also enough energy intake from food should provide for an adequate nutrient and non-nutrient intake. Of the physical activities that can be continued into later life, walking must be one of the most accessible, but it is also true that cultural preferences for other forms of physical activity, for instance, Tai Chi amongst the Chinese, are evident.

### Substance abuse

Smoking (Harris *et al.*, 1988), alcohol (Iber, 1990), medication (Roe, 1983), herbal and nutrient supplements (Wang and Ren, 1988) are among the common lifestyle factors associated with substance abuse.

The smoking habit varies greatly by gender and culture, irrespective of development (Wahlqvist, 1982). Alcohol is uncommonly used in less affluent traditional cultures, especially by women (Wahlqvist *et al.* 1993), although peri-Mediterranean communities are a typical case in point (Kouris *et al.*, 1991). Again, whether herbal or traditional remedies may be used extensively, and with a heritage to draw on, economics and pharmaceutical availability and lack of pressure may limit Western medication and nutrient supplements. Whether, and how well, these abuses are managed, or deleterious consequences avoided, will depend in part on physiological and nutritional reserve capacities.

### Studying the Relationship

The study of nutrition–health relationships in the elderly in the developing world is challenging because of their socio-cultural variation. The Rapid Assessment Procedures (RAP) are a rapid ethnographic method for the assessment of nutrition and health status, with less likelihood of missing the unfamiliar or familiar (Scrimshaw and Hutardo, 1987; Messer, 1991). They allow a better understanding of socio-cultural factors influencing nutrition and health. The use of RAP to study elderly populations in the developing world is an approach where either focus group discussion, or flexible interview and observation, can allow assessment of the impact of both social and nutritional factors on the health of the target group. The application of Rapid Assessment Procedures is inexpensive and effective in studying culturally-diversified, elderly populations (Wahlqvist *et al.*, 1989).

In the case where a standardized study protocol may be difficult to obtain in cross-cultural studies, RAP proves useful in identifying commonality in socio-anthropological determinants of food habits and other lifestyle factors. An example is the elderly populations of similar socio-economic position in the Western Pacific (Andrews *et al.*, 1986), where differences in culture and health status were considered. In the IUNS study on *Food habits in later life* (Wahlqvist *et al.*, 1993), a spectrum of elderly populations differing socio-economically as well as culturally was studied. This latter study can take into account the potential impact of socio-economic development on the nutritional status and health in the elderly in various parts of the world, using a multivariate approach.

## LESSONS FROM AROUND THE WORLD

### The Western Pacific

One of the few studies of a representative sample of elderly people is *Ageing in the Western Pacific: A four-country study*, which was conducted by the World Health Organization Regional Office for the Western Pacific (Andrews *et al.*, 1986). Participating countries were Fiji, the Republic of Korea, Malaysia, and the Philippines. Data are available on the basic demography, health and functional ability, mental health, use of health services, living conditions, way of life, but not on food intake. Many of the variables can be compared with other studies which have subsequently been conducted. These data provided a basic understanding of differences across various developing countries, and highlighted the extent to which socio-cultural factors may affect food habits and practices, food beliefs, nutritional status, and hence the health status of the elderly. For example, family structure and loneliness are explored. How these factors might influence the nutritional status of the elderly in the developing world has yet to be addressed. In a developed society, Horwath (1989) observed that, amongst social factors, living alone had the greatest negative impact on dietary habits and estimated nutrient intake of elderly men.

It is also interesting that in the Western Pacific study, about one-quarter of the total aged population engaged in full- or part-time work, with higher proportions being evident among men and rural dwellers. Those elderly who continue to work are likely to benefit from food intake to match the energy expenditure.

## Meso-America

In Central America, gerontological research has begun to emerge in two countries: Guatemala and Costa Rica. It s a joint initiative between the Centre for Studies of Sensory Impairment, Ageing, and Metabolism (CeSSIAM) in Guatemala and the Institute for Health Research (INISA) in Costa Rica. Some similarities exist between the two Republics. Both are Spanish-speaking countries; both have a largely agrarian society; the majority of the populations of the two nations live on highland plains; and coffee export is a major economic activity. In many ways, however, these two nations could not be more different and divergent. The racial make-up of Costa Rica is largely uniform (*ladinos*). Guatemala, by contrast, has 65 per cent indigenous population with the remaining 35 per cent being *ladinos*. Adult literacy is only 42.4 per cent, whereas Costa Ricans are virtually 100 per cent literate. In terms of health status, there is also a wide gap between the two nations: the infant mortality rate in Guatemala is 71.4 per 1000, whereas in Costa Rica it is 15 per 1000. Guatemala is classified as a less developed country, whereas Costa Rica is a nation in transition to development.

It has been reported that: (1) micronutrient deficiency states exist commonly amongst the elderly of Guatemala, and (2) in terms of body composition, both underweight (deficiency) and overweight/obesity (excess) may be observed in the elderly population of Central America. The state of nutritional excess appears to be more common in Costa Rica than Guatemala (Solomons *et al.*, 1993).

## International Union of Nutritional Sciences (IUNS)

Most studies on the elderly describe the health and functional ability of the elderly and the use of health services. Little information is available on the food habits of elderly people in different countries and cultures and on the impact of presumed lifelong and current eating habits on health in later life. The International Union of Nutritional Sciences (IUNS) committee on Nutrition and Ageing, in conjunction with the World Health Organization (WHO) Global Program for the Elderly, has launched on a programme designed to test key hypotheses in relation to food habits and health status in the elderly in developed and developing countries. The participating centres are:

1. *Australia*
   Aboriginal Australians in Junjuwa, Western Australia aged 55 years and above.
   Anglo-Celtic Melbournians (ACA), aged 70 years and above.
   Greeks in Melbourne (GRK-M), aged 70 years and above.
2. *China*
   Chinese in Rural Tianjin (CTJ-R), aged 70 years and above.
   Chinese in Urban Tianjin (CTJ-U), aged 70 years and above.
   Chinese in Beijing (CBJ), aged 55 years and above.
3. *Greece*
   Greeks in Spata (GRK-S), aged 70 years and above.
4. *Japan*
   Japanese in four districts of Japan, aged 70 years and above.
5. *Philippines*
   Filipinos in Manila (FIL), aged 55 years and above.
6. *Sweden*
   Swedes in Gothenburg (SW), aged 70 years and above.

This study aims to describe present and past food habits, lifestyles, and health status among the aged in developed and developing countries, and to determine to what extent food habits and lifestyle variables, namely, social activity, social network, exercise, activities of daily living, substance abuse, and mental function and well-being may predict the self-perceived and/or medically-defined health status of the elderly. The data provide indicators for further research and evaluation of food–health relationships in developing countries.

## Definition of the 'elderly'

*Chronological age* is the most usual basis of the definition. Geriatric medicine now partitions the young old from the very old with a cut-off point which is progressing with time towards a later and later age. For example, in developed countries, the cut-off point is moving from 70 to 80 years, and even 85 years. In developing countries, the problems often remain that the cohort of the elderly who are over 70 years is small because of low life expectancy. For this reason, studies on health in the aged have been inclined to consider the upper decile or quintile of the representation graph of the aged. This may mean including people as young as 45 or 50. A limitation of this approach is ascertaining the base of the population pyramid. For example, the proportion of people who are elderly can vary from society to society, depending on the birth rate and mortality rate amongst the young. An alternative for developing countries would be to consider life expectancy at birth, and examine those who had reached an age approximating at least a certain number of years into this life expectancy.

A separate issue is the question of identifying the aged on the basis of their biology as distinct from their chronology. But dependable markers of *biological age* are few, and there is insufficient agreement on how these should be synthesized to score biological age (Steen, 1993). Particular examples of biological age include voice analysis (Linville and Fisher, 1985), skin change in non-ultraviolet exposed areas (Holman, 1984), and steroid hormone profile (Walford, 1986).

It also needs to be said that *social age* has great significance, meriting documentation in studies of nutrition–health in later life. An example of the determination of women's age by society comes from a consideration of Chinese women who, after menopause, wear a different attire, namely, trouser-type garments rather than the customary dress. Thus, in a study of the aged and their food habits, it may be necessary to identify societal markers of age. Again, the number of generations that have already succeeded one—children, grandchildren, great-grandchildren—creates a common definition of age. Take an individual who has a child early in life—this young parent is more likely to be regarded as elderly than if he were childless. The designation of 'grandparent' itself connotes aged!

## Methodology

Low literacy levels limit the use of self-administered questionnaires. The interviewer and other observers therefore play an important role in obtaining valid data. Preparative work using RAP has proven valuable in becoming familiar with a community, in minimizing the impact of preconceived notions, and ensuring that key points are not missed or neglected (Scrimshaw and Hutardo, 1987).

## Illustrative data

Cross-cultural comparisons suggest distinct differences between study centres in terms of *food intake*, self-assessment of health, and body mass index. Legume intake was 10 g per day in old-old men (80 years and above) in rural Tianjin, and 182 g per day in their urban counterparts (Fig. 4.2). Similar variation in daily food intake has been observed in rural–urban comparisons. Further, cross-cultural differences in intakes of certain food products were observed. For example, Beijing Chinese young-old men (those between 55 and 70 years) consumed about 10 g of milk and milk products per day and, by contrast, the Swedish young-old men (those aged between 70 and 79 years) consumed over 400 g per day (Fig. 4.3).

Self assessment of *health* also showed differences amongst study centres. Most of the elderly Greeks in Melbourne claimed to be in good health (56 per cent in young-old women to 76 per cent in young-old men), while a relatively small percentage of the elderly rural Tianjin Chinese made the same claim (7.6 per cent in young-old women to 20 per cent in very old men) (Fig. 4.4). On the other hand, if we look at comparisons on *body mass index* (BMI), elderly Greeks in Melbourne have the highest BMI (27 in old-old women to 31 in young-old men), while the elderly rural Tianjin Chinese have the lowest BMI (18 in old old men to 21 in young-old women) (Fig. 4.5).

## CONCLUSIONS AND DIRECTIONS FOR THE FUTURE

Research on nutrition and health in old age has so far received low priority whilst the focus has been on problems of nutrition in childhood. Increasing longevity now establishes the need for more attention to problems of nutrition and health in the elderly. The return on *future research* into the changing nutrition–health relationships in later life with development will be greater if the likely problems are specifically addressed. For example, dependence on staples and a restrictive range of food; micronutrient deficiencies such as those of iron and zinc; osteoporosis (not only because of fracture risk, but also because of bone nutrient storage); immunodeficiency which may increase the prevalence of infectious and neoplastic diseases; abdominal obesity leading to diabetes and macrovascular disease. Such research needs to be under way before a *nutrition policy for the elderly* is settled, unless the limitations spelt out in the policy, and research is promoted as part of the policy.

There is a need to encourage growth in *geriatric nutrition as a subject for medical education* at the undergraduate and postgraduate levels. This will foster rapport between the elderly and their health care providers in a way that will be conducive to competent preventive and health care.

In *community health programmes*, community health workers will need to be equipped to advise and educate the population at large on

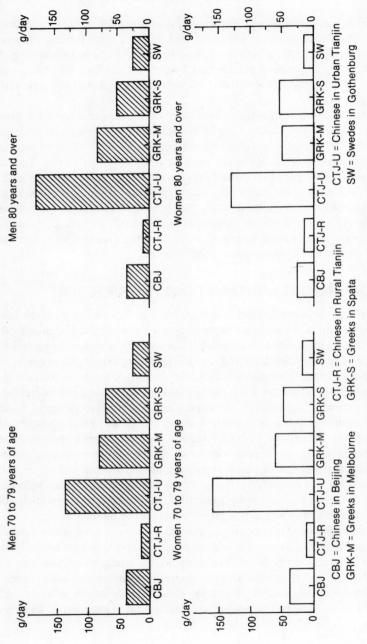

**Fig. 4.2.** Legume intake (g/day) by IUNS study centres (by age group, by gender)

CBJ = Chinese in Beijing     CTJ-R = Chinese in Rural Tianjin     CTJ-U = Chinese in Urban Tianjin

GRK-M = Greeks in Melbourne     GRK-S = Greeks in Spata     SW = Swedes in Gothenburg

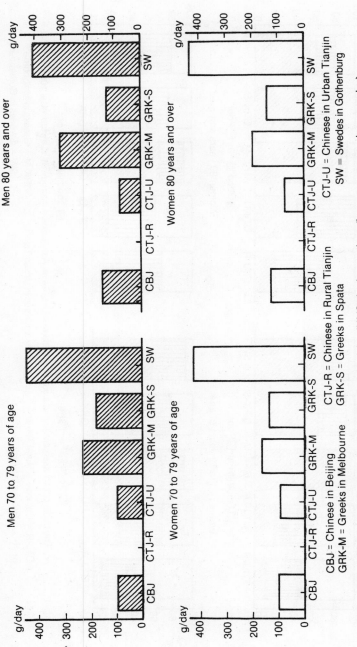

**Fig. 4.3.** Milk and dairy product intake (g/day) by IUNS study centres (by age group, by gender)

CBJ = Chinese in Beijing    CTJ-R = Chinese in Rural Tianjin
GRK-M = Greeks in Melbourne   GRK-S = Greeks in Spata
CTJ-U = Chinese in Urban Tianjin
SW = Swedes in Gothenburg

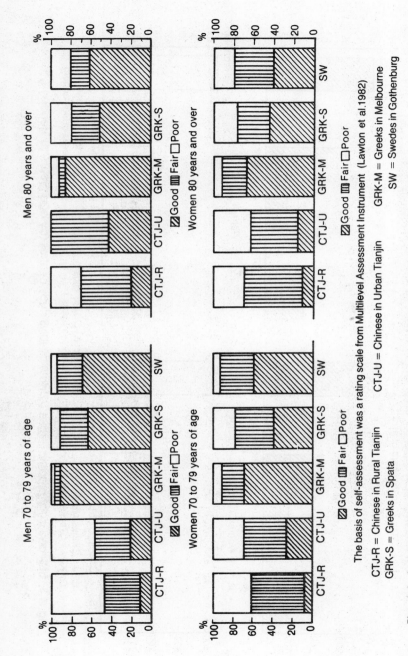

**Fig. 4.4.** Self-assessment of health by IUNS study centres (by age group, by gender)

The basis of self-assessment was a rating scale from Multilevel Assessment Instrument (Lawton et al.1982)

CTJ-R = Chinese in Rural Tianjin    CTJ-U = Chinese in Urban Tianjin

GRK-S = Greeks in Spata         GRK-M = Greeks in Melbourne

SW = Swedes in Gothenburg

Men 80 years and over

Women 80 years and over

Men 70 to 79 years of age

Women 70 to 79 years of age

Good   Fair   Poor

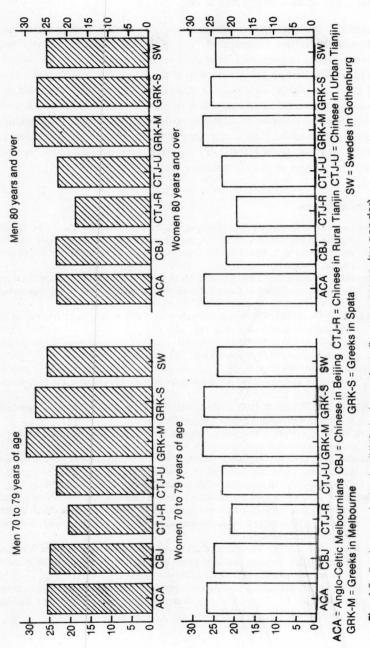

**Fig. 4.5.** Body mass index by IUNS study centres (by age group, by gender)

ACA = Anglo-Celtic Melbournians CBJ = Chinese in Beijing CTJ-R = Chinese in Rural Tianjin CTJ-U = Chinese in Urban Tianjin
GRK-M = Greeks in Melbourne GRK-S = Greeks in Spata SW = Swedes in Gothenburg

culturally sensitive and economically-viable healthy eating and related physical activities. Therapeutic nutrition and physical activity programmes may be preferred, or at least be treated as a prelude and adjunct to pharmacotherapy. Early detection of those at high risk in communities of older people through documentation of their nutritional status will facilitate prevention and correction of nutritionally-related health problems. For this purpose, instruments to assess food–health relationships, such as those of the IUNS, may need to be acquired at the local level by health workers. Such efforts will increase the prospects of the aged as valued members of their community and their nation.

## REFERENCES

Andrews, G. R., Esterman, A. J., Braunac-Mayer, A. J., and Rungie, C. M. (1986). Ageing in the Western Pacific. A four-country study. Western Pacific Reports and Studies No. 1, World Health Organization, Regional Office for the Western Pacific, Manila.

Arnauld, J., Alarcon, J. A., and Immink, M. D. C. (1990). Food security and food and nutrition surveillance in Central America: The need for functional approaches. *Food and Nutrition Bulletin*, **12**(1), 26–33.

Astrand, P. O. (1968). Physical performance as a function of age. *Journal of the American Medical Association*, **205**, 729–33.

Bjorntorp, P. (1990). Abdominal obesity and risk. *Clinical and Experimental Hyper-Theory and Practice*, **A12**(5), 783–94.

Briggs, D. and Wahlqvist, M. L. (eds). (1988). *Food Facts. The Complete No-Fads-Plain-Facts Guide to Healthy Eating*. Melbourne, Penguin Books Australia Ltd, 22.

Bucht, G. and Sandman, P. O. (1990). Nutritional aspects of dementia, especially Alzheimer's disease. *Age and Ageing*, **19**, S32–36.

Chandra, R. K. (1990). The relation between immunology, nutrition, and disease in elderly people. *Age and Ageing*, **19**, S25–31.

Chandra, R. K. (1990a). Nutrition is an important determinant of immunity in old age. In: Prinsley, D. M. and Sanstead, H. H. (eds). *Nutrition and Aging: Progress in Clinical Biological Research*, Alan R. Liss Inc, New York, **326**, 321–34.

Chandra, R. K., Joshi, P., Au, B., Woodford, G., and Chandra, S. (1982). Nutrition and immunocompetence of the elderly: Effect of short-term nutritional supplementation on cell-mediated immunity and lymphocyte subsets. *Nutrition Research*, **2**, 223–32.

Davidson, M. B. (1979). The effect of aging on carbohydrate metabolism: A review of the English literature and a practical approach to the diagnosis of diabetes mellitus in the elderly. *Metabolism*, **28**(6), 688–705.

Davies, L. (1990). Socioeconomic, psychological and educational aspects of nutrition in old age. In: Steen B. (ed). *Nutrition and Aging. Age and Ageing*, **19**(Supplement No. 1), S37–42.

Dontas, A. S., Marketos, S. G., and Papanayiotou, P. (1972). Mechanisms of renal tubular defects in old age. *Postgraduate Medical Journal*, **48**, 295.

Duchateau, J., Delepesse, G., Vrijens, R., and Collet, H. (1981). Beneficial effects of oral zinc supplementation on the immune response of old people. *The American Journal of Medicine*, **70**, 1001–4.

Dupin, H. (1974). Factors influencing eating patterns in the developing world. *Impact of Science on Society*, **24**(2), 145–50.

Duthie, H. L., and Bennett, R. C. (1963). The relation of sensation in the anal canal to the functional anal sphincter: A possible factor in anal incontinence. *Gut*, **4**, 179–82.

Ferro-Luzzi, A., Scaccini, C., Taffese, S., Aberra, B., and Demeke, T. (1990). Seasonal energy deficiency in Ethiopian rural women. *European Journal of Clinical Nutrition*, **44**(Suppl 1), 7–18.

Flint, D. M., Wahlqvist, M. L., Smith, T. J., and Parish, A. E. (1981). Zinc and protein status in the elderly. *Journal of Human Nutrition*, **35**, 287–95.

Friedman, M., Green, M. F., and Sharland, E. (1969). Assessment of hypothalamic pituitary adrenal function in the geriatric age group. *Journal of Gerontology* **24**(9), 292–6.

Gopalan, C. (1992). *Nutrition in Developmental Transition in South-East Asia*, World Health Organization, Regional Office for South-East Asia, New Delhi.

Griffin, R. M. (1975). Social structure and urban disease: Need for a broader base for health planning and research. *Urban and Social Change Review*, **8**(1), 15–20.

Hage, B. H. H. (1992). Food habits and cardiovascular health status in adult Melbourne Chinese. Thesis, Department of Medicine, Monash University.

Harris, T., Cook, E. F., Garrison, R., Higgins, M., Kannel, W., and Goldman, L. (1988). Body mass index and mortality among nonsmoking older persons. The Framingham heart study. *Journal of the American Medical Association*, **259**, 1520–4.

Herbert, V. (1990). Nutritional anaemias in the elderly. In: Prinsley, D. M. and Sanstead, H. H. (eds). *Nutrition and Aging: Progress in Clinical Biological Research*, Alan R. Liss, New York, **326**, 203–27.

Holman, C. D. J., Amstrong, B. K., Evans, P. R., Lumsden, G. J., Dallimore, K. J., Meehan, C. J., Beagley, J., and Gibson, I. M. (1984). Relationship of solar keratosis and history of skin cancer to objective measures of actinic skin damage. *British Journal of Dermatology*, **110**, 129–38.

Horwath, C. C. (1989). Socio-economic and behavioral effects of the dietary habits of elderly people. *International Journal of Biosocial and Medical Research*, **11**(1), 15–30.

Iber, F. L. (1990). Alcoholism and associated malnutrition in the elderly. In: Prinsley, D. M. and Sanstead, H. H. (eds). *Nutrition and Aging: Progress in Clinical and Biological Research*, Alan R. Liss Inc, New York, **326**, 157–73.

James, W. P. T., Ferro-Luzzi, A., and Waterlow, J. C. (1988). Definition of chronic energy deficiency in adults. Report of a Working Party of the International Dietary Energy Consultative Group. *European Journal of Clinical Nutrition*, **42**, 969–81.

Kahne, H. (1981). Women and social security: Social policy adjusts to social change. *International Journal of Aging and Human Development*, **13**(3), 195–208.

Khandker, Shahibur R. (1989). Improving rural wages in India. Policy, Planning, and

Research Working Paper 276. World Bank, Population and Human Resources Department, Washington, D.C., USA.

Kouris A., Wahlqvist, M. L., Trichopoulus, A., and Polychronopoulus, E. (1991). Use of combined methodologies in assessing food beliefs and habits of elderly Greeks in Greece. *Food and Nutrition Bulletin*, **13**, 139–44.

Lawton, M. P., Moss M., Fulcomer, M., Kleban, M. H. (1982). A research and service oriented multilevel assessment instrument, *Journal of Gerontology*, **37**, 91–9.

Lee, H. P. (1992). Diet and cancer—Some results from Singapore. *Asia Pacific Journal of Clinical Nutrition*, **1**, 43–6.

Leeds, M. (1981). Inflation and the elderly: A housing perspective. *Annals of the American Academy of Political and Social Science*, **456**, 60–9.

Lindeman, R. D., Tobin, J., and Shock, N. W. (1985). Longitudinal studies on the rate of decline in renal function with age. *Journal of the American Geriatrics Society*, **33**, 278–85.

Linville, S. E. and Fisher, H. B. (1985). Acoustic characteristics of women's voices with advancing age. *Journal of Gerontology*, **40**(3), 324–30.

Messer, E. (1991). International Conference on Rapid Assessment Methodologies for Planning and Evaluation of Health Related Programmes: Interpretative summary. *Food and Nutrition Bulletin*, **13**(4), 287–92.

Meydani, S. N., Barklund, M. P., Liu, S., Meydani, M., Miller, R. A., Cannon, J. G., Morrow, F. D., Rocklin, R., and Blumberg, J. B. (1990). Vitamin E supplementation enhances cell-mediated immunity in healthy elderly subjects. *American Journal of Clinical Nutrition*, **52**, 557–63.

Ogawa, Naohiro *et al.* (1982). Japan's limits to growth and welfare. *Population Ageing in Japan: Problems and Policy Issues in 21st Century*. Tokyo, Nihon University.

Olsen, R. B., Olsen, J., Gunner-Svensson, F., and Waldstrom, B. (1991). Social network and longevity. A 14-year follow-up study among elderly in Denmark. *Social Science and Medicine*, **33**(10), 1189–95.

Pobee, J. O. M. (1980). The status of cardiovascular disease in the setting of disease of environmental sanitation and hygiene and malnutrition: The West African (Ghana) experience. In: Lauer, R. M. and Shekelle, R. B. (eds). *Childhood Prevention of Atherosclerosis and Hypertension*, New York, Raven Press.

Powles, J. (1992). Changes in disease patterns and related social trends. *Asia Pacific Journal of Clinical Nutrition*.

Riggs, B. L. and Melton III, L. J. (1986). Involutional osteoporosis. *The New England Journal of Medicine*, **314**(26), 1676–86.

Roe, D. A. (ed). (1983). *Geriatric Nutrition*. Prentice-Hall Inc, New Jersey, 155–73.

Roe, D. A. (1984). Nutrient and drug interactions. *Nutrition Reviews*, **42**(4), 141–54.

Rogers, R. G. (1989). Life expectancy in less developed countries: Socio-economic development or public health? *Journal of Biosocial Science*, **21**(2), 245–52.

Rolls, B. J. and Phillips, P. A. (1990). Aging and disturbances of thirst and fluid balance. *Nutrition Review*, **48**(3), 137–44.

Saltzman, R. L. and Peterson, P. K. (1987). Immunodeficiency of the elderly. *Reviews of Infectious Diseases*, **9**(6), 1127–39.

Sandman, P. O., Adolfsson, R., Nygren, C., Hallmans, G., and Winblad, B. (1987). Nutritional status and dietary intake in institutionalized patients with

Alzheimer's disease and multiinfarct dementia. *Journal of the American Geriatrics Society*, **35**, 31.

Scrimshaw, S. C. M. and Hutardo, E. (1987). Rapid assessment procedures for nutrition and primary health care: Anthropological approaches to improving programme effectiveness. UCLA Latin American Center, Los Angeles, California, USA.

Shephard, R. J. (1986). Nutrition and the physiology of aging. In: Young, E. A (ed). *Contemporary Issues in Clinical Nutrition: Nutrition, Aging, and Health*, 1–23, Alan R. Liss Inc, New York.

Silverstein, M. and Bengtson, V. L. (1991). Do close parent–child relations reduce the mortality risk of older parents? *Journal of Health and Social Behaviour*, **32**(4), 382–95.

Smith, E. L., Smith, P. E., and Gilligan, C. (1988). Diet, exercise, and chronic disease patterns in older adults. *Nutrition Reviews*, **46**(2), 52–61.

Solomons, N. W. (1992). Nutrition and aging: Potentials and problems for research in developing countries. *Nutrition Reviews*, **50**(8), 1–8.

Solomons, N. W., Lacle, A., Mazariegos, M., and Mendoza, I. (1993). Spontaneous gerontological research initiatives in Central America. In: Wahlqvist, M. L., Davies, L., Hsu-Hage, B., Kouris-Blazos, A., Scrimshaw, N., Steen, B., and van Staveren, W. (eds). *Food Habits in Later Life: Cross-Cultural Approaches*. United Nations University Press.

Steen, B. (1988). Body composition and aging. *Nutrition Reviews*, **46**(2), 45–51.

Steen, B. (1993). Blood pressure, biochemical analyses and cutaneous microtopography. In: Wahlqvist, M. L., Davies, L., Hsu-Hage, B., Kouris-Blazos, A., Scrimshaw, N., Steen, B., and van Staveren, W. (eds). *Food Habits in Later Life: Cross-Cultural Approaches*. United Nations University Press.

Thompson, E. N., and William, R. (1965). Effect of age on liver function with particular reference to bromsulphalein excretion. *Gut*, **6**, 266–9.

Wahlqvist, M. L. (1982). Social toxicants and nutritional status. In: Jelliffe, E. F. P. and Jelliffe, D. B. *Adverse Effects of Foods*. New York, Plenum Press, 227–38.

Wahlqvist, M. L., Davies, L., Hsu-Hage, B. H-H., Kouris-Blazos, A., Scrimshaw, N., Steen, B., van Staveren, W. (eds). (1993). *Food Habits in Later Life: Cross-Cultural Approaches*. United Nations University Press.

Wahlqvist, M. L., and Kouris, A. (1990). Trans-cultural aspects of nutrition in old age. In: Steen, B. (ed). *Nutrition and Aging. Age and Ageing*, **19**(supplement No. 1), S43–52.

Wahlqvist, M. L., Kouris, A., Gracey, M., and Sullivan, H. (1989). Rapid assessment procedures and a study of the food habits and health of elderly aboriginal Australians: Junjuwa community. In: Kim, W. Y., Lee, Y. C., Lee, K. Y., J. S. J, Kim, S. H. (eds). *Proceedings of the 14th International Congress of Nutrition*, vol. II, 231–2.

Wahlqvist, M. L., Lo, C. S., and Myers, K. (1989). Food variety is protective against macrovascular disease in type 2 diabetes. *Journal of the American College of Nutrition*, **8**(6), 515–23.

Walford R. (1986). *The 120 Year Diet: How to Double your Vital Years*, New York, Simon and Schuster.

Wang, Z. G. and Ren, J. (1988). Pharmacology and toxicology of traditional Chinese medicines—A historical perspective. In: McLean, A. J. and Wahlqvist, M. L. (eds). *Current Problems in Nutrition Pharmacology and Toxicology*, London, John Libbey, 44–9.

Walker, A. (1981). Towards a political economy of old age. *Ageing and Society*, **1**(Part 1), 73–94.

Webster, S. G. P. (1980). Gastrointestinal function and absorption of nutrients. In: Exton-Smith, A. N., Caird, F. I. (eds). *Metabolic and Nutritional Disorders in the Elderly*. Bristol, John Wright, 86–9.

Wilcox, G., Wahlqvist, M. L., Burger, H., and Medley, G. (1990). Oestrogenic effects of plant food in postmenopausal women. *British Medical Journal*, **301**, 905–6.

World Development Report. (1990). *Poverty*. Oxford, Oxford University Press.

World Health Organization. (1989). *Program for Research on Ageing*: *Executive Summary*, WHO, Geneva.

World Health Organization. (1990). *Diet, Nutrition, and the Prevention of Chronic Disease*. Report of a WHO Study Group, WHO, Geneva.

# 5

# Effects of Gender of Head of Household on Women's and Children's Nutritional Status

EILEEN KENNEDY, PAULINE PETERS, AND
LAWRENCE HADDAD

## INTRODUCTION

A major debate in the literature on Women in Development revolves
around the issue of whether economic development benefits or harms
women in developing countries. A part of this debate focuses on the
differential effects of macro-economic policies on women-headed
households. An increasing number of households in both developing and
developed countries are headed by women (Folbre, 1991). Policymakers
are concerned that these women-headed households are poorer and
potentially less likely to benefit from development policies.

The purpose of this chapter is to summarize what is known about
trends in the number of female-headed households and the vulnerability
of these households to poverty. Particular attention is paid to identifying
the health and nutritional status of women and children in different
household structures, including various categories of women-headed
households.

## DEFINING A FEMALE-HEADED HOUSEHOLD

Households are the most common unit of analysis in survey research,
including censuses. The concept of 'head of household' was introduced
into census surveys in order to avoid double counting. However, the

head of household is also a concept that has historically implied greater authority, including economic authority, within the household structure.

The literature is clear that in surveys in developing countries in which there is self-reporting of headship, households will almost invariably report a male head of household, even if the person concerned is absent for extended periods (ICRW, 1988). Until recently, female-headed households in many countries were seen as synonymous with households without a single male member. But as Folbre (1991) points out, aside from its political connotations, this conventional terminology is asymmetrical, defining a household as female-headed only if there is no man present. However, the term 'male-headed' is applicable whether or not there is an adult female in the household, reflecting the scant value given to women's domestic labour as an input to household maintenance.

As far back as 1978 (Buvinic and Youssef, 1978), researchers highlighted the fact that the conventionally-used definition of female-headed household (that is, manless) was too limiting. Legally, female-headed or *de jure* female-headed households were only one type, and not necessarily the most common type, of female-headed household. Many women have the day-to-day responsibility of maintaining households and these households are therefore *de facto* women-headed. Unfortunately, the category of *de facto* female-headed households is rarely included in census surveys.

More recently, a number of researchers have begun to question the assumption that headship implies economic responsibility. The concept of 'female-maintained' household has been used to signify a household in which a disproportionate share of income and/or work effort is provided by the woman.

The assumption of headship in most definitions is that the designed head of household has more authority in decision-making within the household structure. Thus, in *de jure* and *de facto* female-headed households, women have more authority in household decisions than do women in male-headed or jointly-headed households.[1] Similarly, using the alternative definitions of female-maintained households, the assumption is typically that if women contribute more work hours, or a higher percentage of household income, then they will have more control than men over household decision-making.

---

[1] Jointly-headed households, although a classification of headship, are only infrequently given in surveys with self-reported headship.

The newer definitions of headship, which are emerging, are useful in helping us 'unpack' some of the assumptions underlying the traditional approaches used in defining household structure. The definitions that are ultimately used will affect the number of households that are identified and, equally important, the characteristics of those households.

Demographic and social changes have resulted in increases in the number of female-headed households. In the United States, Canada, and Europe, divorce, separation, and widowhood have resulted in an increasing number of residential units headed by women (ICRW, 1988). Folbre (1991) points out that modernization has had a contradictory impact on women. On the one hand, an increasing number of women are entering the labour force, providing the potential for more economic independence and political participation. Yet Folbre also highlights the fact that 'studies of women's workday in developed countries show that these gains have been purchased at a very high price, an extremely long workday and increased responsibility for the financial support of their children'.

The number of female-headed households is also increasing in developing countries, but the reasons differ. In Latin America, a combination of rural-to-urban migration, primarily by single women, and an increase in adolescent fertility has led to a rise in female-headed households (CEPAL, 1985; Economic Commission for Latin America and the Caribbean, 1991). Louise Fox's (1989) continuing work in Brazil suggests that female headship is increasing, with 20 per cent of all urban households being female-headed. In Africa, the migration of men in search of wage employment has led to an increase in *de facto* female-headed households. Asia has had less of a tradition of migration of females from rural to urban areas; this is, in part, reflected in the low percentage of female householders in Asia. Yet there is evidence of an increasing number of female-headed households in South India. A recently completed study of Gender and Poverty in India reports that 35 per cent of households below the poverty line are headed by women (World Bank, 1991).

The concern with these statistics is not simply that the number of female-maintained, or female-headed households, is growing but that these households are perceived to be poorer and/or less likely to be helped by typical economic development policies adopted by most countries. The next section explores the evidence between gender of head of household and poverty.

## ARE FEMALE-HEADED HOUSEHOLDS POORER?

Many donors tend to believe that poverty is more common in female-headed households. However, it is clear from the previous section that female-headed households are not a homogeneous entity. Data in Table 5.1 for Ghana, Kenya, and Malawi show that the relationship between household income and gender of head of household is mediated, in part, by the type of female-headed household.

For Kenya, a simple comparison between male-headed and the all-female head of household category shows that income per capita is significantly higher in the male-headed households. However, when female-headed households are disaggregated in *de jure* and *de facto* female-headed households, a different pattern emerges: there is no significant difference between male- and *de jure* female-headed households in

**Table 5.1** Demographic characteristics and expenditure patterns of households in Kenya, Malawi, and Ghana

| Country/<br>Household type | | Demographic characteristics | | |
| --- | --- | --- | --- | --- |
| | | Household<br>size | Dependency<br>ratio | Expenditures<br>per capita |
| Kenya[**] | | | | |
| Male | | 9.55 | 1.23[*] | 2854.0[*] |
| Female: | Total | 9.10 | 1.34[*] | 2561.0[*] |
| | *de jure* | 8.62 | 1.24 | 2736.0 |
| | *de facto* | 10.09 | 1.54[*] | 2200.0[*] |
| Malawi[**] | | | | |
| Male | | 6.26 | 1.28 | 81.1[*] |
| Female: | Total | 5.64 | 1.76 | 71.7[*] |
| | Migrants | 6.21 | 2.49 | 114.1[*] |
| | *de jure* | 5.10 | 1.55 | 63.5[*] |
| | *de facto* | 5.90 | 1.68 | 59.7[*] |
| Ghana[†] | | | | |
| Male | | 6.92 | 1.28 | 44,201.0 |
| Female: | All females | 5.29 | 1.81 | 43,115.5 |
| | *de jure* | 5.31 | 1.83 | 43,181.0 |
| | *de facto* | 5.31 | 1.52 | 45,352.0 |

In Kenya shillings (per annum) for Kenya; kwacha (per 10 months) in Malawi; and cedis (per month?) for Ghana
[**] Taken from Kennedy and Peters (1992)
[*] Significantly different than male-headed households at p<0.05
[†] Taken from Kennedy and Haddad (1994)

income per capita. However, *de facto* female-headed households are significantly poorer than male-headed households in the same community.

The data for Malawi are even more intriguing. Here, similar to the findings for Kenya, male-headed households have a significantly higher expenditure per capita as compared with the category of all-female-headed households. *De facto* female-headed households in the Malawi sample were separated into two distinct groups: the typical *de facto* households and migrant households, where a *de facto* female head receives remittances from a male member working specifically in South Africa.

However, when male-headed households are compared with different types of female-headed households, the patterns change. The richest and poorest household types in the Malawi sample are female-headed. Migrant households receiving remittances from South Africa are the wealthiest, and the *de facto* are the poorest. Migrant households have expenditures per capita that are significantly higher than male-headed households, and *de facto* female-headed households have income levels that are significantly lower than male-headed households.

The data for Ghana in Table 5.1 indicate that women-headed households are, on average, no poorer than male-headed households. There are no significant differences, on average, between male-headed, *de jure* female-headed, and *de facto* female-headed income levels in Ghana.

To the question, 'Are female-headed households poorer than male-headed households?', the answer is, 'not always'. However, the data presented in Table 5.1 represent African case studies only, and it may be misleading to extrapolate the findings to female-headed households in other areas of the world. Several authors have highlighted the fact that female-headed households have had more of a tradition in Africa. Even in sheltered, Islamic societies, such as the Hausa in Nigeria, Polly Hill (1969) noted that matrilineal descent patterns led to the existence of independent producers which has, historically, led to the formation of women-headed households.

Female-headed households arising as a result of traditional patterns sanctioned by society may be less likely to be poor (CEPAL, 1985). Examples are evident in the migrant households in Malawi, in Ghana, and in some women-headed households in Kenya.

In many of the studies reviewed by Gupta (1989), female-headed households tended to be over-represented among the poor. This is more true for Latin America and Asia than it is for Africa. In Latin America, poorer female-headed households are more likely to be found in urban areas, whereas in Africa, female-headed households are more prevalent in rural areas.

From a policy perspective, what is more useful than simply knowing the number and trends in female headedness is an understanding of the links between poverty and female headship. Some common factors contribute to the higher probability of poverty in female-headed households.

First, although female-headed households tend to have a smaller household size than male-headed households,[2] they have a higher dependency ratio, as shown in Table 5.1. The income earnings of a fewer number of adults have to be shared by a larger number of dependents.

Secondly, the average earnings of adult females tend to be lower than for adult males. A part of this is attributed to the lower levels of education, on average, for women as compared to those for men. This female/male education gap was identified in the recent World Bank Report on Poverty (World Bank, 1990). Data from Peru indicate that a shorter education span for women is a significant, negative determinant of lower earnings (Tienda and Salazar, 1980).

Many women have time constraints related to child care and home responsibilities which increase the probability of working in the informal sector where earnings tend to be lower. However, data controlling for education, working in the informal sector, and number of children still indicate that women earn less than men (Buvinic, 1990).

Finally, there is a large body of evidence that indicates that women have less access to credit and other financial services than men (Buvinic, 1990; Barnes, 1983).

The contribution of these factors varies by country and by region. However, the combination of these variables contributes to a higher probability of poverty in female-headed households in many parts of the developing world.

## NUTRITIONAL STATUS OF CHILDREN FROM FEMALE-HEADED HOUSEHOLDS

Because the number of female-headed households has been increasing throughout the developing world, and since these households in many cases are poorer, national level policymakers and donors are concerned that this trend may have a negative effect on children. Data from Kenya, Ghana, and Malawi were used to look at the linkages between different types of female-headed households and pre-schooler nutritional status.

[2] Again, there are exceptions to this rule.

Table 5.2 presents some of the results. In Kenya, pre-schoolers from male-headed households are significantly more likely to be stunted and have a low weight-for-age in comparison with children from the aggregate of all female-headed households. Possibly more surprising is the finding that the lowest income, *de facto* female-headed households have lower levels of pre-schooler malnutrition (based on weight-for-age) than children from male-headed households; 14.6 per cent of pre-schoolers from *de facto* female-headed households are moderately to severely malnourished (below −2.0 Z-score for weight-for-age) as against 18.6 per cent of children in male-headed households.

Similar results are indicated for Malawi: in the lowest income, *de facto* female-headed households, weight-for-age less than −2.0 Z-scores is 20.9 per cent as against 28.4 per cent in male headed households. Pre-schoolers from *de facto* female-headed households are also less likely to be stunted than pre-schoolers from male-headed households.

Curiously, pre-schoolers from the highest income, migrant female-headed households in Malawi do no better nutritionally than children from male-headed households. It is, therefore, not gender of the head of household *per se* that automatically imparts this beneficial effect on the nutritional status of pre-schoolers.

In Ghana, there is no significant difference between the nutritional status of pre-schoolers of male-headed households and that of different types of female-headed households. These descriptive data lead to the conclusion that even in Africa the relationship between headship and pre-schooler nutritional status is not consistent. We begin to get a hint of an explanation of the findings from the data presented in Table 5.2.

In Kenya, there is a tendency for children from female-headed households to be sick for a shorter period; for example, they have shorter bouts of diarrhoea. None of these differences, however, are statistically significant.

In both Kenya and Malawi, the proportion of household calories obtained by the pre-schooler is higher in the lower income, *de facto* female-headed households. For example, pre-schoolers from migrant female-headed households in Malawi, despite their higher incomes and higher levels of household caloric adequacy, do not themselves have the highest pre-schooler energy intake nor the best nutritional status in comparison with children from other types of households. On the contrary, the proportion of calories obtained by children in these higher-income, migrant, female-headed households is below even that in male-headed households. This is due, in part, to the types of extra calories acquired,

**Table 5.2** Nutritional status and morbidity of pre-schoolers

| | Kenya** | | | | Malawi** | | | | | Ghana† | | | |
| --- | --- | --- | --- | --- | --- | --- | --- | --- | --- | --- | --- | --- | --- |
| | Male | Female | | | Male | Total | Migrants | Female | | Male | All female | | |
| | | Total | de jure | de facto | | | | de jure | de facto | | | de jure | de facto |
| Z-scores: | | | | | | | | | | | | | |
| Weight–age | −1.07* | −0.87* | −0.84 | −0.91* | −1.45 | −1.38 | −1.53 | −1.23 | −1.42 | −1.15 | −1.18 | −1.17 | −1.24 |
| Height–age | −1.66* | −1.41* | −1.40 | −1.44 | −2.41 | −2.31 | −2.64 | −2.16 | −2.24 | | | | . |
| Weight–height | −0.06 | −0.01 | 0.01 | −0.06 | 0.06 | 0.05 | −0.06 | −0.16 | −0.04 | | | | |
| Per cent with Z-scores less than −2: | | | | | | | | | | | | | |
| Weight–age | 18.6 | 15.5 | 16.0 | 14.6 | 28.4 | 23.5 | 36.0 | 17.7 | 20.9 | 21.9 | 19.6 | 19.6 | 20.0 |
| Height–age | 39.9 | 32.8 | 33.1 | 32.1 | 62.3 | 55.9 | 64.0 | 55.9 | 51.2 | | | | . |
| Weight–height | 1.9 | 4.6 | 4.5 | 4.8 | 0.9 | 0.0 | 0.0 | 0.0 | 0.0 | | | | |
| Per cent less than −2 | 18.6 | 15.5** | 16.0 | 14.6** | 28.4 | 24.2 | 36.0 | 19.4 | 20.9 | 22.0 | 19.8 | 15.4 | 20.0 |
| Bottom tercile | 19.9 | 15.9 | 19.7 | 9.8 | 31.3 | 25.6 | 0.0 | 27.8 | 28.6 | 23.0 | 20.3 | 15.3 | 37.5 |
| Middle tercile | 20.6 | 13.2 | 7.7 | 20.7 | 40.7 | 13.0 | 40.0 | 0.0 | 8.3 | 22.3 | 21.5 | 15.2 | 17.7 |
| Top tercile | 15.6 | 17.1 | 17.5 | 15.8 | 10.6 | 30.3 | 43.8 | 14.3 | 20.0 | 20.3 | 16.9 | 15.9 | 15.0 |

| | Kenya** | | | | Malawi** | | | | | Ghana† | | |
|---|---|---|---|---|---|---|---|---|---|---|---|---|
| | Male | Female | | | Male | Migrants | Female | | | Male | All fe-male | |
| | | Total | de jure | de facto | | Total | | de jure | de facto | | de jure | de facto |
| **Per cent of total time:** | | | | | | | | | | | | |
| I 11 | 28.63 | 27.80 | 27.82 | 27.75 | 21.80 | 22.80 | 19.00 | 27.20 | 21.10 | | | |
| I 11 with diarrhoea | 4.14 | 4.00 | 3.97 | 4.05 | 1.84 | 1.90 | 1.63 | 2.39 | 1.63 | | | |
| Child/household caloric adequacy | 0.66 | 0.67 | 0.64 | 0.72 | 1.31 | 1.37 | 1.19 | 1.36 | 1.48 | | | |

** Taken from Kennedy and Peters (1992)
† Taken from Kennedy and Haddad (1994)
* Significantly different from male-headed households at p<0.05

namely, meat and other expensive foods, that often do not directly increase pre-schooler caloric intake. Similarly, in Kenya, *de jure* households (whose expenditure levels are about equal to male-headed households) also allocate a slightly lower proportion of total calories to their children than do male-headed households. These findings suggest that, as household incomes increase, there is not necessarily a direct one-to-one effect on the caloric adequacy of pre-schooler diets.

The reason for higher allocation of calories to children in lower income, *de facto* female-headed households is not clear. It could be that, given limited resources, investment of income in the form of food for children brings the highest return from among the few alternative investment options of poorer households. By investing in their children, these poorer households may best be able to insure their long-term security. Such an explanation is consistent with the data presented above on the declining share of expenditure on food as incomes increase. It is also consistent with the observation that male-headed households, and wealthier female-headed households, spend a higher proportion of income on other productive assets, such as inputs into cash crop production, including fertilizers. The consumption needs of adult household members and investments in land, hired labour, and other productive resources may compete with children's consumption for a share of the budget in households where incomes are sufficiently high to allow those additional investments.

Another explanation for the negative relationship between household income and the proportion of calories accruing to children may be that, at higher levels of income, money is spent on more expensive calories rather than more calories *per se*. Children simply may not share proportionately in those additional, more expensive calories. This certainly appears to be the case in the Malawi households. Moreover, the failure of an increase in income to positively affect child nutrition may be due to the type and timing of income. Migrant households in Malawi, for example, receive, on average, a much higher income than other female heads, but, one, the sizeable remittances may incline the recipients to spend on items other than the daily requirements of pre-schoolers and, two, migrant remittances may not last more than a few years in some families.[3] Finally, the Malawi study suggests that where cash incomes

---

[3]Recruitment of migrant workers for South Africa has now been stopped by the Malawi government. A current study being undertaken by Peters of the same Malawian households as described in this article aims to assess the effects of this change on income and consumption of former migrant households.

are higher, and where these allow higher levels of expenditure, the resources allocated to appropriate feeding of young children is *not* proportionately higher. This would suggest that additional efforts have to be made in education and in providing the means (such as more effective weaning foods or energy-efficient cooking technologies) for directing increased incomes towards the vulnerable pre-schoolers.

Finally, the Kenya example also points to the importance of nurturing behaviour in determining the quality of child nutrition. According to a detailed, ethnographic study conducted as part of the Kenya research (Rubin, 1988), female-headed households often feed their pre-school children more frequently than male-headed households. Analyses have shown that a child's caloric adequacy increases in proportion to the number of daily meals (for example, Kennedy, 1989).

In the case of *de jure* households, the higher prevalence of disease and lower proportion of calories allocated to children, as compared with *de facto* households, may partly reflect the relationship of the household head to the child members. In Kenya, and to a lesser extent in Malawi, many of the female household heads in *de jure* households are the grandmothers of children in the household. In terms of the impact on child health and nutrition, the fact that a woman heads the household may be less important than the relationship between the household head and the child members. The degree of authority that mothers wield in decisions with regard to their own children's well-being may have an overriding importance in allocations of income for additional health care or food for children. Inter-generational conflicts over the value of modern health and nutrition practices that limit their adoption may also affect child well-being.

In Kenya, the findings on pre-schooler nutritional status are more dramatic for the lowest income tercile; children in the lowest income, *de facto* female-headed households are significantly less likely to be moderately and severely malnourished than children from male-headed households. Clearly, it is not female-headedness *per se* that leads to better nutrition for children, but the intersection between income and gender of head.

The findings from Kenya, namely, that it is the children in the lowest income, *de facto* female-headed households that do significantly better than pre-schoolers from low-income, male-headed households, are similar to the findings reported by Johnson and Rogers (1991) for the Dominican Republic. It was only in the lowest quartile of income that the per cent of total household income earned by the mother was significant-

ly associated with children's nutritional status. In the upper three quar-
tiles of income, there was no differential effect of maternal income on
pre-schooler nutritional status. The studies from Kenya and the Dominican Republic suggest that distributional patterns of income (and possibly
time) at very low levels of income in these female-headed households
are a key factor in working to the advantage of children's nutrition.

## NUTRITIONAL STATUS OF WOMEN IN FEMALE-HEADED HOUSEHOLDS

Not so long ago, women's nutrition was given attention only as it affected infant and child nutrition. It is only very recently that Maternal
and Infant Nutrition has been relabelled Woman and Infant Nutrition by
a number of donors. It is not surprising, then, that the amount of information available on the nutritional and health status of non-pregnant,
non-breast-feeding women is limited; and there is almost none available
on the relationship between gender of head of household and women's
nutrition.

Some nutritional status data disaggregated by gender of head of
household are presented for women in Kenya (Table 5.3). The data are
categorized not only by gender of household head but by terciles of
income per capita. Nutritional status as measured by body mass index
(BMI) is significantly higher for women in all female-headed households combined than for women from male-headed households. Women
in *de jure* and *de facto* headed households (all income terciles combined)
have a higher BMI than women from male-headed households. These
differences are not significant but are influenced partly by the small
sample size in some of the cells.

Presence in a *de facto* female-headed household does not have a positive effect on women's nutritional status. Part of the explanation is the
level of energy intensity of women's activities as shown in Table 5.3. It
is commonly observed that in male-headed and *de jure* female-headed
households, as household income increases, the energy expenditure of
women decreases. However, in *de facto* female-headed households, as
household income increases, women continue to experience a high level
of energy expenditure. Time spent in work is significantly higher for
women from *de facto* female-headed households than for women from
*de jure* female-headed households in the middle income tercile.

These issues need to be probed further, but they point again to the

**Table 5.3** Selected women indicators, by gender of head of household, by household income per capita tercile (1=lowest tercile)

| Indicator | Male | All Female | All Female de jure | All Female de facto | All |
|---|---|---|---|---|---|
| **Body Mass Index** | | | | | |
| 1 | 22.41 | 22.84 | 22.45 | 23.44 | 22.49 |
| 2 | 22.12 | 22.40 | 22.70 | 21.67 | 22.16 |
| 3 | 22.13 | 22.89 | 22.70 | 23.68 | 22.25 |
| All terciles | 22.21[a] | 22.72[a] | 22.62 | 22.94 | 22.30 |
| N | 819 | 174 | 122 | 52 | 993 |
| **Total energy expenditure/day** | | | | | |
| 1 | 2562.12 | 2561.94 | 2554.48 | 2573.59 | 2562.08 |
| 2 | 2552.82 | 2573.57 | 2556.90 | 2623.61 | 2556.49 |
| 3 | 2498.19 | 2498.96 | 2459.88 | 2676.59 | 2498.33 |
| All terciles | 2538.02 | 2546.98 | 2523.31 | 2606.35 | 2539.73 |
| N | 879 | 207 | 148 | 59 | 1086 |
| **Per cent total time ill** | | | | | |
| 1 | 18.82[b] | 21.62 | 25.28[b] | 17.54 | 19.44 |
| 2 | 23.81[b] | 18.55 | 11.58[b] | 29.20 | 23.01 |
| 3 | 23.27 | 23.65 | 21.95 | 29.98 | 23.33 |

(*Continued*)

**Table 5.3** (Continued)

| Indicator | Male | All Female | All Female | | All |
|---|---|---|---|---|---|
| | | | *de jure* | *de facto* | |
| All tercilles | 21.96 | 21.38 | 20.43 | 22.97 | 21.85 |
| N | 786 | 176 | 110 | 66 | 962 |
| Non-leisure time (hours/day) | | | | | |
| 1 | 10.41 | 10.61[b] | 10.84[b] | 10.23 | 10.45 |
| 2 | 10.49 | 10.44 | 9.99[c] | 11.80 | 10.48 |
| 3 | 10.05 | 9.34[b] | 9.00[b] | 10.96 | 9.93 |
| All terciles | 10.32 | 10.19 | 9.95 | 10.81 | 10.30 |
| N | 947 | 219 | 159 | 60 | 1166 |
| Per cent share of income | | | | | |
| 1 | 29.93[b] | 38.62 | 42.81 | 34.75 | 31.64 |
| 2 | 27.72 | 34.86 | 37.63 | 31.12 | 28.79 |
| 3 | 22.12[a,b,c] | 45.78[a] | 60.14[c] | 28.22[c] | 24.23 |
| All terciles | 26.68[a,b] | 38.56[a] | 44.02[c] | 32.47 | 28.44 |
| N | 644 | 112 | 59 | 53 | 756 |

Source: IFPRI South Nyanza Survey, 1985/87

[a] The difference between male-versus female-headed household within tercile group is significnt at the 0.05 level
[b] The difference *across terciles* within each gender of head of household category is significant at the 0.05 level
[c] The difference from among male-, *de jure* female-, and *de facto* female-headed household within each tercile group is significant at the 0.05 level

importance of not treating female-headed households as a homogeneous entity.

## CONCLUSIONS

Since the mid-1970s, the number of women-headed households has been increasing in both industrialized and developing countries. The limited definitions that have been used to categorize women-headed households probably result in an underestimation of the number of women-headed and women-maintained households.

Until recently, little information on the effects of economic policies on the health and nutritional status of women and children from women-headed households was available. Given the growing importance of female-headed and women-maintained households, it would be useful for policymakers to have some system for monitoring the effect of policies and programmes on women and children in different types of household structures.

Some issues that need consideration include:

— What are the specific coping strategies used to ensure food security, health, and nutritional status in female-headed versus male-headed households? How do changing economic policies enhance or negate these strategies?
— Very often our comparisons of health and nutritional outcomes in male-headed versus female-headed households are restricted to short-term phenomena. What are the longer-term welfare consequences of membership in a female-headed household?
— Gender of the head of household is known to change, particularly in Africa. Are some of the positive health and nutrition effects observed in certain types of female-headed households maintained in the longer term?
— Is poverty in female-headed households transferred to the next generation? Why or why not?

## REFERENCES

Barnes, Carolyn (1983). *Rural Africana*, **41**, 15–16.
Buvinic, Myra (1990). The feminization of poverty. In: *Women and Nutrition*, ACC/SCN, Geneva.
Buvinic, Myra and Youssef, Nadia (1978). Women-headed households: The ignored factor in development planning. Report for the U.S.A.I.D., Office of Women in Development, Washington, D.C..

CEPAL (1985). *Analysis Estadistico de la Situacion de la Mujer en paises de America Latina a Traves de las Encuentras de Hogares.* Mimeo.

Economic Commission for Latin America and the Caribbean (1991). *The Vulnerability of Households Headed by Women: Policy Questions and Options for Latin America and the Caribbean.* Social Development Division, Women and Development Unit, Santiago.

Folbre, Nancy (1991). *Women on Their Own: Global Patterns of Female Headship.* Population Council/ICRW Working Paper Series, Washington, D.C.

Fox, Louise (1989). Poverty, female-headed families, and the welfare of children and youth in Brazil: Preliminary evidence and research agenda. Paper presented at the Population Council/ICRW Seminar Series on Determinants and Consequences of Female-headed Households.

Gupta, Geeta (1989). Female-headed households, poverty, and child welfare. Paper presented at the Population Council/ICRW Seminar Series on Determinants and Consequences of Female-headed Households.

Hill, Polly (1969). Hidden trade in Hausaland. *Man,* **4.**

ICRW (1988). Women-headed households: Issues for discussion. Paper prepared for the Joint Population Council/ICRW Seminar Series on the Determinants and Consequences of Female-headed Households.

Johnson, Katherine and Rogers, Beatrice (1991). Effects of female headship in Dominician Republic. *Social Science and Medicine.*

Kennedy, Eileen (1989). *The Effects of Sugarcane Production on Food Security, Health, and Nutrition in Kenya: A Longitudinal Analysis.* IFPRI Research Report 78. International Food Policy Research Institute, Washington, D.C., USA.

Kennedy, Eileen and Haddad, Lawrence (1994). Are pre-schoolers from female-headed households less malnourished?: A comparative analysis of results from Ghana and Kenya. *Journal of Development Studies.*

Kennedy, Eileen and Peters, Pauline (1992). Influence of gender of health of household on food security, health, and nutrition. *World Development,* **20**(8), 1077.

Rubin, Deborah (1988). Ethnographic research in a sugarcane-growing community in Kenya. Final report submitted to U.S.A.I.D., Office of Policy and Program Coordination, Washington, D.C.

Tienda, Marta and Salazar, Sylvia (1980). Female-headed households and extended family formation in rural and urban Peru. University of Wisconsin, Madison Center for Demography and Ecology, Madison, Wisconsin. Mimeo.

World Bank (1990). *Poverty and Development.* World Development Report, Washington, D.C., USA.

World Bank (1991). *Gender and Poverty in India.* Washington, D.C., USA.

# 6

# Communication and Nutrition Education

## MOHAMED El-GHORAB AND MAMDOUH GABR

## INTRODUCTION

Malnutrition, 'the silent killer', causes widespread distress, especially in developing countries. Malnutrition is caused by one or more of a complex web of different factors—physiological, personal, social, cultural, economical, and political—at a specific time for a given individual.

Food shortage may be a leading cause of malnutrition in over-congested regions. But deeper analysis of the situation reveals that an insufficient food supply is not solely responsible for malnutrition in the world. Ignorance and illiteracy, prevailing attitudes to and superstitions about food play an equally important role in the spread of malnutrition among a given population.

Several studies have revealed that the success of nutrition education programmes in changing nutrition behavioural patterns and in reducing the prevalence of malnutrition depends on the collaboration between professional communicators and nutritionists throughout the design and implementation of the intervention. It has rightly been said: 'Teach a mother to be healthy and she will teach the rest of mankind.' Unfortunately, the role of women as health providers and nutritional caretakers has been given scant respect.

It must be recognized, however, that nutrition-related behaviour is more difficult to change than many other health-related behavioural patterns. Therefore, special attention must be given to the process of assessment, planning, development, and to pre-testing messages, delivery, and continued programme monitoring in making timely changes.

## HISTORICAL BACKGROUND

Communication, a process as old as man, is the transfer of ideas or information from one person to another. When two persons meet they pass on and receive information automatically, and this occurs even when they do not speak the same language. Nutrition education evolved from primarily face-to-face instruction in the 1950s and 1960s to a social marketing approach in the 1970s, which incorporated market research methodologies and mass media. In the 1980s, new research techniques, which have been useful in identifying behaviour susceptible to modification and in formulating specific messages were applied, whereas earlier programmes focused on promotion. The new programmes began to regard 'products' as an idea, for instance, breast-feeding. The concept of 'price' was also expanded to include not only money but also other costs in opportunity and time. Another development has been the growing emphasis on prevention (and hence nutrition education) which accompanied the introduction of the primary health care concept in 1978 (Lediard, 1991).

## DEFINITION

Nutrition education is the process by which people gain the knowledge, attitude, confidence, and skills necessary for developing good dietary practices.

## EFFICIENCY

It is now generally accepted that nutrition education is cost-effective. However, despite the major contribution made in the field, the efficiency of nutrition education programmes has been questioned. Disappointing reports on nutrition education effects namely, that negligible impact has been made on nutrition-related behaviour, have sparked debate among nutrition educators. Furthermore, it is argued that fortifying food or increasing people's income will improve the nutritional status more than nutrition education programmes. Unfortunately, many nutrition education programmes, which were not geared to socio-economic or political situations in the country, helped to encourage such sentiments. Also, efforts in nutrition education over the past few years have been limited to interpersonal communication techniques, using simple media such as various forms of printing material. It is becoming clear that a nutrition education programme that uses a multimedia approach, including face-to-face communication, other traditional communication means, and mass media technology, will be more fruitful. Moreover, illiteracy, lack of infrastructure, and inappropriate use of expensive technology have resulted in minimal nutrition education at the village level, with difficulty in instruction and disappointing results. On the other hand, opting for mass media such as radio and television, which has a wide range of use, has proved effective in health education.

While dissemination of information through newspapers, pamphlets, posters, radio, and television has positively educated target audiences and moderately influenced attitudes, this strategy has had little effect on changing behaviour patterns. Changing behaviour, rather than disseminating knowledge, must be the clear intention of a programme for effective results (Cerqueira, 1991).

Finally, it should be recognized that nutrition education is distinctly different from other types of health education in that improved nutrition requires sustained and repeated individual endeavour. Furthermore, changes in eating patterns have less tangible and less immediate pay-offs than other preventive measures such as immunization.

## LEARNING AND TEACHING

There is some confusion with respect to the terms 'teaching' and 'learning'. Teachers believe that if they *teach* a subject, the audience will *learn* it. This is not always the case. Moreover, in programmes aimed at changing behaviour, information should not be confused with education. Education in food and nutrition entails the adoption of better practices. The acquisition of knowledge does not in itself necessarily lead to different behaviour; it requires motive and intention. People may know about nutrients and about balanced diet without applying this knowledge in their daily life. The process by which people adopt new ideas is complex and involves several steps: awareness, interest, evaluation, trial, and finally, adoption. Nutrition education cannot be considered complete until the new practice is actually adopted.

Learning is an active process, and education is more successful when the learner takes part in the process (Richie, 1969).

## PLANNING NUTRITION EDUCATION PROGRAMMES

The steps to be followed in planning a nutrition education programme are the same as those applicable to the solving of problems. However, some other factors need to be considered in planning and carrying out nutrition education programmes. These are the specific groups of people you want to reach, and the kind of information you want to impart. According to the *Nutrition Handbook for Community Workers in the Tropics* (1986) these steps are as follows: After identifying problems, decide on the central problem. Suggest causes and plan a course of remedial action after discussing all possible solutions. Carry out the plan, which should revolve around the selected solution, and finally evaluate the results.

## Principles for Successful Nutrition Education Programmes

A number of key principles could be generalized to all nutrition education programmes regardless of scale, or type of media used. These include:

1. A comprehensive and systematic approach to conceptualize, implement, and evaluate the programme. A complete understanding of the target group, including its behaviour, attitudes, and political and environmental constraints, is essential for a successful communication programme. The objective of the education programme must be realistic. We should remember that nutrition education cannot solve all nutrition problems.

   Although a comprehensive media approach is essential, it is equally urgent to revise the strategy based on the feedback from monitoring and evaluation. A substantial number of people cannot be drawn to new ideas if the educators are restricted to a few methods and materials that were learned at a specific time, in a specific set of circumstances. It should be remembered that there is more than one way to achieve a goal.

2. Another criterion for a successful programme is *the support of policy-makers or decision-makers and health care officials*. This support is critical for programme sustainability and the success of a nutrition education programme. The need to visualize problems in their order of priority and select those that can be resolved is also essential.

   Social marketing is an effective model for the development of nutrition education programmes. Social marketing is not a theory in the formal sense since it does not attempt to explain causes. It is a model that orders and structures information and procedures, and as such, it allows for the incorporation of a number of theories. Choice of theory—for example, motivation, information processing, or family dynamics—should depend on the problem addressed.

3. The use of the multimedia approach, including face-to-face communication and other traditional methods, is a key factor in determining the success of a programme. Television messages have tremendous power in changing behaviour, but they by themselves cannot bring about sustainable change. For example, studies have revealed that the use of television and radio is more effective in communicating nutrition information than radio alone. Clear visualization appears to be crucial in communicating with target groups, especially illiterate people. Educational programmes must use an entertaining, non-didactic approach, and they need to be flexible enough to revise the strategy based on feedback from monitoring and evaluation.

## METHODOLOGIES

The several methods used in nutrition education include group discussion and decision-making group activities; demonstration of method followed by discussion and practice; demonstration and discussion of results achieved by members of the community; role playing and drama; interviews (Richie, 1969).

More didactic methods such as lectures, speeches, mass contacts through media such as film, radio, and television programmes, and leaflets and posters are effective when they are used in combination with more personal methods of communication which espouse an exchange of ideas and encourage audience participation.

### Group Discussion and Decision-making

Evidence suggests that group discussion leading to a decision may be a fruitful method in modifying social behaviour. When attitudes are frankly examined during a discussion, a person is obliged to acknowledge them and to recognize them in the light of other people's comments. The pressures that build up within a group help to influence the individual members. The feeling of belonging and the support of others make it easier for a person to resolve to change his attitudes and to adhere to his resolutions. In group decision, the members are jointly supporting one or another conflicting alternative. For these reasons, decisions taken by a group after a thorough discussion are more likely to be carried out than those made by individuals.

## Drama

Dramatizing a story or situation is a useful educational tool. Plays and songs are popular with school children. Puppet plays were used in a variety of educational campaigns. Shadow plays, another form of puppetry, are acted behind a translucent screen, using cut-out, jointed figures on sticks or strings, and cut-out cardboard props and scenery.

## Role Playing

Role playing is a specialized form of acting, particularly suitable for staff and students. It entails acting the various roles in a real-life situation in order to instil a deeper understanding of its implications and the relationships involved in it.

## Mass Media

Mass media can be a powerful tool for promoting health. Television is a major source of role models for a wide range of health-related behaviour. Research indicates that there is a great potential for people to imitate televised behaviour if this is easy to execute, is performed by attractive models, and either generates positive reinforcement or is reacted to in a natural way.

In spite of its importance, television has not been used widely in many developing countries, where it is most needed. In most of these countries, where the problem of malnutrition is most acute, audio-visual facilities are totally unavailable or strictly limited. Mass media can be gainfully utilized to explain certain diseases as well as principles of hygiene, along with a few basic facts about nutrition. Faulty habits, rather than unavailability of food, are the major cause of malnutrition in some countries, and an informal mass media campaign elucidating the basic principles of nutrition can help to reduce the prevalence of malnutrition in these countries.

Although radio has the advantage of widespread coverage, it has not yet shown promising results in communicating nutrition information. Radio messages have not yet gripped audience attention.

Mass media, however, should not replace more traditional, interpersonal communication. The vehicle of communication should make use of all existing systems and methods to convey the messages.

## Media selection

Although certain media are better suited to certain messages, audiences, and circumstances, there does not seem to be any generally superior medium or media mix. The selection of appropriate media depends on:

(a) The skills and attitudes of the audience in relation to the available media.
(b) The size and dispersion of the audience. Are they a small select group or most of the population? Are they dispersed or concentrated?
(c) The local resources, both financial and technical.
(d) The nature of the responses we want the audience to be able to make and the nature of the reinforcement we want to be able to give.

## The Message

From the data collected, we can develop a series of messages. In developing the message the following points are essential (Anderson, 1984):

(a) The message should be clear and easily understood. Simple, common words should be used.
(b) The message should be tailored to the recipients' lifestyles, values, tradition, and culture.
(c) The method used to send the message must match the ability of the target group.
(d) The message should suggest changes which the group can carry out.
(e) There should be no contradiction between the message and what the community workers say in other sectors.

## Pre-testing the message

The message should be tested and evaluated. Pre-testing messages with a small number of people helps to ensure that a message is well suited to the target group. After testing, you may need to edit the message, or alter the method or material used.

## Communicating the message

The message could be communicated by means of several methods—the spoken word, the written word, and visually—either separately or

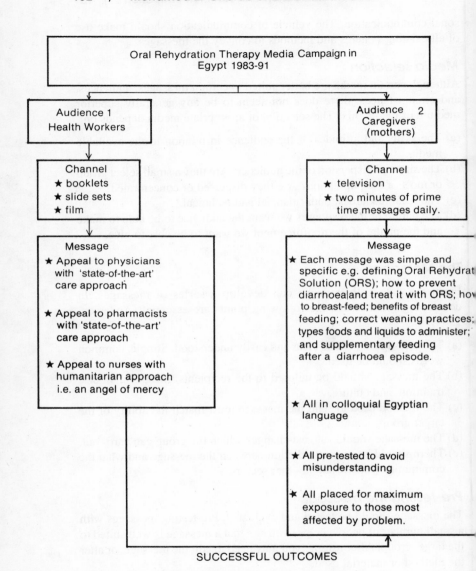

**Fig. 6.1** A summary of the target audiences and messages selected and developed for nutrition communication in Egypt

together. For example, the spoken word can be combined with movement, as in television, films, or plays. Before choosing a method of communicating messages, we should make sure that it suits the people, their circumstances, and the problem to be solved.

A plan of action for communicating messages also needs to be developed as part of the whole nutrition education programme, such as

— The number of times the message is repeated.
— The method used.
— The time of the message.
— The effect of the message.

Short, focused, specific messages are better understood by individuals of limited education. The content of the messages for the public should be approved by medical authorities, and should not be weighted with too much information.

Several successful nutrition communication programmes in various parts of the world have significantly changed specific nutrition and food-related behaviour patterns. These programmes used the social marketing model to guide their design and implementation.

## CASE STUDY 1

### Nutrition Behaviour Change in Egypt (El Kamel, 1991)

In this programme, a modern, social-marketing theory was applied to a specific problem in Egypt, namely, oral rehydration therapy (Fig 6.1).

A baseline community survey of 2100 persons estimated that 90 per cent of Egyptian households viewed television, 95 per cent of all households owned radios, and the majority of the sample population was illiterate. Mothers did not believe in the Oral Rehydration Solution (ORS) and did not know how to treat diarrhoea.

Accordingly, the programme set two objectives:

1. Use social marketing to educate the public about nutrition needs during diarrhoea; and
2. to produce results, distribute and promote the use of ORS. The target audience included mothers and health providers.

The messages were carefully designed, the content being a blend of emotion and information. The knowledge of ORS rose from zero to 99 per cent in seven years; and the use of ORS rose from 50 per cent to 79 per cent in six years. About 300,000 children were saved during this period.

It is concluded that this campaign succeeded for the following reasons:

— the media were used effectively;
— the indigenous culture was closely observed, respected, and incorporated into the programme;
— sociological and anthropological research findings were well integrated;
— all the steps of the social marketing theory were applied.

## CASE STUDY 2

## Nutrition Education in Health Centres in Egypt (El-Ghorab, 1987)

The National Nutrition Survey of Egypt, which was carried out in 1978, showed a high prevalence of chronic undernutrition among pre-school children. Anaemia was prevalent among 38 per cent of the pre-schoolers, and 22 per cent of pregnant mothers and lactating women. These alarming figures directed attention towards the fact that preventive measures should be initiated to combat these problems. One of the most important measures was the introduction of nutrition education in health centres.

The project, which began in 1979 by a grant-agreement between the Ministry of Health and the Catholic Relief Services utilizing a USAID fund, aimed to develop a nutrition education programme that would strengthen the food and nutrition services delivered through the health infrastructure in Egypt. The project sought to achieve that purpose largely through teaching mothers attending MCH centres about nutrition, hygiene, and child care. The nutrition messages were directed mainly towards pre-school child nutrition and the best use of food aid offered at these centres as well as the use of growth charts. The developed curriculum included information on basic nutrition, balanced diet, breast-feeding, weaning practices, growth charts, and nutrition during specific illnesses. The project equipped an educational kitchen in the centres in addition to providing audio-visual materials.

The Nutrition Institute in Cairo was assigned the responsibility of project implementation and training. Six regional supervisors were in charge of the project activities in the different governorates. Later the

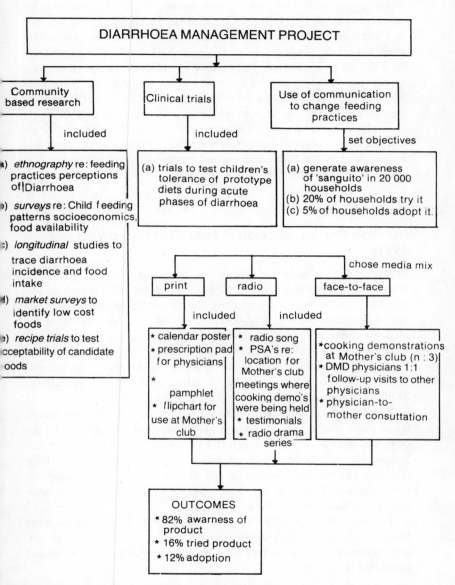

**Fig. 6.2** A summary of the research process used to develop the messages in the Diarrhoea Management Project in Peru

Ministry of Health took over implementation while the Nutrition Institute retained responsibility for the training activities.

More than 600 health centres participated in the nutrition programme in almost all the governorates of Egypt, and more than 2000 staff from the Ministry of Health received training in nutrition. Two manuals, one for nurses and the second for doctors, and one training video film were developed. Mothers learned the proper use of child feeding. The use of the manual by the nurses was, however, minimal. The growth charts were also not used by all the centres. as the medical staff had to cope with the onerous curative activities. Experience made it amply clear that involvement of the policy-makers and health officials in the education programme is essential.

## CASE STUDY 3

### Nutrition Communication in Peru (Cabanero Versoza, 1991)

In a campaign to introduce special dietary formula for young children with diarrhoea in Peru, the communication mix included messages targeted to physicians and those giving child care. Radio messages in the native language were widely accepted. In addition, the messages included a radio-drama series on treatment for diarrhoea. Print materials were developed for physicians. Professional seminars were organized for them, and there were one-to-one visits to ensure their support and cooperation. Flip charts were used during cooking demonstrations. Traditional media, including a local theatre, were also used.

Results showed that radio reached 87 per cent of the population, home clubs reached 25 per cent of households, print messages, 19 per cent, and doctors or nurses reached 5 per cent. Sixteen per cent of the households tried the new products, and 12 per cent adopted them. Those who heard of the new product only via the radio had the lowest adoption rates, whereas those who heard the message via the radio plus another source registered the highest adoption rates.

The programme also revealed that nutritionists and communicators have complementary and supportive roles to play throughout the design and implementation of interventions aimed at changing nutrition-related behaviour (Fig. 6.2).

## CASE STUDY 4

## Nutrition Education in India (Agarwal and Udipi, 1989)

The programme aimed at educating mothers on health and nutrition issues. It was conducted by a voluntary agency, the Sophia Rotary Medical Centre. Functionaries in this programme were illiterate women. Health workers living in the same area as the mothers were responsible for health education. The health and nutrition education classes given to the mothers were followed by routine home visits. Sessions included the use of films and other audio-visual aids, demonstrations, and competitions.

The programme covered the following topics: the importance of breast-feeding, supplementary and weaning foods, balanced diet, diet during pregnancy and lactation, immunization, and sanitation and hygiene.

The programme was deemed successful in changing the attitudes to and practices in respect of children's health and nutrition, and proved an extremely valuable tool in alleviating the malnutrition that may arise as a result of delayed weaning. One of the lessons learned is that it is essential to have personnel who are motivated and, as far as possible, able to grasp the problems of the beneficiaries. Also, the ratio of beneficiaries to health workers must be kept within manageable limits.

## CONCLUSIONS

Nutrition-related behaviour is more complicated to change than many other health related behaviour patterns. Nutrition behavioural change must be subtle, and often requires an entire series of messages leading gradually to the desired change.

Effective and affordable nutrition education programmes can be designed and implemented in various countries and circumstances to address wide-ranging needs. These programmes are effective when professional communicators and nutritionists work closely together throughout the design and implementation of the intervention programme.

Principles for successful nutrition programmes are:

(a) The programme should depend on a comprehensive and systematic approach to conceptualize, implement, and evaluate it.
(b) Support of policy-makers and health care workers is essential.

face communication, other traditional communication means, and mass media technology.

Social marketing can provide a model for guiding the development of a nutrition communication programme. Products (or targeted behaviour and message strategy) of a social marketing programme can rarely be transferred to other situations, unlike the decision-making process which is adaptable.

## REFERENCES

Agarwal, Momta and Udipi, Shobha (1989). The impact of nutrition education on child-feeding practices among low-income urban Indian mothers. *Food and Nutrition Bulletin*, **11**, 32.

Anderson, J. (1984) The ABC model for developing communication to change behaviour. In: Tanphaichitr, V., Dahlan, W., Suphakarn, V., and Valyasevi, A. (eds). *Human Nutrition, Better Nutrition, Better Life*. Proceedings of the Fourth Asian Congress of Nutrition held in Bangkok, Thailand, 1983, Aksornsmai Press, Bangkok, 115–23.

Cabanero Versoza, Cecilia. Nutrition interventions in Peru and Nigeria. In: Achterberg, Cheryl (ed). *Effective Nutrition Communication for Behaviour Change*. Report of the Sixth International Conference of the International Nutrition Planners Forum, Paris. Office of Nutrition, U.S.A.I.D., Washington D.C., 12–14.

Cerqueira, M. T. (1991). Nutrition education: A review of the nutrient-based approach. *Food, Nutrition and Agriculture*, **1**, 30.

El-Ghorab, M. (1987). Nutrition education in maternal and child health centres. Workshop on Intersectorial Collaboration for Nutrition Promotion, Egyptian Nutrition Institute/WHO, Cairo.

El Kamel, Farag (1991). The Egyptian experience with nutrition behaviour change. In: Achterberg, Cheryl (ed). *Effective Nutrition Communication for Behaviour Change*. Report of the Sixth International Conference of the International Nutrition Planners Forum, Paris. Office of Nutrition, U.S.A.I.D., Washington D.C., 6–8.

Lediard, M. (1991). Keynote address. In: Achterberg, C. (ed). *Effective Nutrition Communication for Behaviour Change*. Report of the Sixth International Conference of the International Nutrition Planners Forum, Paris. Office of Nutrition, U.S.A.I.D., Washington D.C., 3–4.

*Nutrition Handbook for Community Workers in the Tropics*. (1986). Macmillan.

Richie, J. (1969). *Learning Better Nutrition*. Food and Agriculture Organization, Rome.

# 7

# Nutritional Effects of Structural Adjustment in Sub-Saharan Africa

DAVID E. SAHN

## INTRODUCTION

During the 1980s, most countries in sub-Saharan Africa began adjusting their economic policies in response to unsustainable imbalances whereby aggregate demand exceeded aggregate supply, as manifested in unsustainable balance of payments and budget deficits. The process of adjustment, broadly speaking, involved a series of macro-economic and sectoral policy changes; these included devaluation of the exchange rate; restructuring of government expenditures and related fiscal restraint; monetary discipline and rationalization of interest rates as well as reforming (and sometimes shrinking) the structure and role of the state and state-run institutions, including public enterprises that engage in agricultural input and product marketing, the government-run health and education system, and other institutions, such as the banking sector and financial markets.

While the process of reform has been considered crucial to restoring growth to faltering African economies, much skepticism about the social impact was voiced, especially during the early stages of adjustment during the mid-1980s. In particular, the potentially deleterious nutritional consequences of economic adjustment were given considerable attention, as summarized in the respective statements of the Deputy Executive Director of UNICEF and Secretary General of the United Nations:

As it mostly operates at the moment, adjustment policy . . . transmits and usually multiplies the impact on the poor and vulnerable. The result, as shown in many countries, is rising malnutrition in the short run . . . (Richard Jolly, 1985)

. . . the implementation of structural adjustment programs has given rise to general concerns. . . . Their human and social costs have often been seen as out of proportion with their real or intended benefits. The most vulnerable population groups, in particular women, youth and disabled and the aged, have been severely and adversely affected. . . . Access to food has become more difficult for large segments of the population, with the result that malnutrition has increased, particularly among children, infants and pregnant women. (Javier Perez de Cuellar)

These are compelling statements of concern over the nutritional effects of structural adjustment. In fact, they ignited a further examination of the impact of adjustment on household living standards, and raised the more fundamental issue as to the appropriateness of the entire gamut of economic adjustment. While research continues on the effect of adjustment on poverty, food security, and nutrition, a sizeable body of literature and experience has been gained over the past few years to inform the debate on the impact of adjustment on households. This will be discussed in the remainder of the chapter, in order to examine whether the early hypothesis of the harmful effects of adjustment on nutrition was correct, and what can, and has been done to alleviate such concerns.

More data are available on the nutrition problems in Africa's urban areas than in its rural regions. In addition, the impact of adjustment in urban areas is more palpable, both because the cities are more acutely affected by state policy, and because the state, in turn, is more attentive to the city-dwellers who exert a disproportionate influence over the government's survival. Nonetheless, we will try to avoid too much of an urban bias in our discussion. This is critical because levels of chronic undernutrition are worse in rural areas, as is evident from the few available nationally representative sample surveys of nutrition (Table 7.1). This, coupled with the fact that Africa's population remains predominantly rural, comprising 72 per cent of the population in 1989 and an even higher percentage in poorer countries that tend to have more malnutrition, suggests a rural focus, despite the fact that the problem of urban malnutrition may indeed worsen commensurate with the rapid pace of urbanization.

Our analysis is organized as follows. A simple conceptual framework for understanding the mechanisms and pathways through which adjustment affects nutrition is followed by a discussion on whether state disengagement from delivering social services has imperilled the nutrition of vulnerable groups. Then the focus moves to the nutritional effects of

**Table 7.1** Indicators of chronic malnutrition in selected African countries

| Country | Survey year | Chronic undernutrition | |
|---------|-------------|------------------|-----------------|
| | | Rural (%) | Urban (%) |
| Cameroon | 1977 | 22.4[†] | 15.7[†] |
| Cote d'Ivoire | 1985 | 18.4[*] | 11.3[*] |
| | 1986 | 19.4[*] | 11.2[*] |
| Ghana | 1987 | 34.8[*] | 22.0[*] |
| | 1988 | 22.8[†] | 12.3[†] |
| Liberia | 1976 | 20.2[†] | 13.8[†] |
| Sierra Leone | 1977 | 26.6[†] | 13.8[†] |
| Togo | 1977 | 20.5[†] | 11.4[†] |
| Uganda | 1988–89 | 46.3[*] | 25.6[*] |
| Zimbabwe | 1988 | 33.6[*] | 14.3[*] |

Sources: Ghana: Alderman (1990); Cote d'Ivoire: Sahn (1990); Cameroon, Liberia, Togo, and Sierra Leone: Alderman (1989); Uganda: (1989); Zimbabwe: DHS (1989)

[*]  Children below –2 Z-scores of reference height-for-age
[†]  Children below 90 per cent of reference height-for-age

changes in the structure and functioning of markets, with particular attention to shifts in relative prices and incomes, and their effect on consumers and producers. Next, we deal with the issue of time use and gender roles, how they may be affected by structural adjustment and the consequent impact on nutrition, and proceed to discuss the role of social funds and compensatory programmes to respond to, and prevent, harmful consequences of adjustment. Finally, we conclude with a presentation of issues and concerns in need of further study and action.

## CONCEPTUAL FRAMEWORK

Before tackling the effects of economic adjustment on nutrition, there is a need to delineate between reforms that fall in the domain of stabilization and those in the field of structural adjustment. In the case of the former, reference is primarily to short-run crisis management through constraining aggregate demand. More precisely, stabilization does not endeavour to alter the rules and institutions that are operative in the economy. Rather, a combination of monetary and fiscal restraints, as well as other policies such as exchange rate realignment, tend to reduce the sum of consumption, government spending, and investment. These measures are therefore contractionary or demand-reducing. The main link to long-term economic growth is the contention that movement toward balance-of-payments equilibrium is a prerequisite to an economic environment that is conducive to prosperity.

In contrast, structural adjustment refers to efforts aimed primarily at medium- and long-term improvements in economic efficiency through rationalizing resource allocation, including factors of production. The rules of the game by which economic agents operate are altered, and institutional structures changed. As such, relative prices, the terms of exchange, returns to factors of production, and so forth are affected in an effort to engender a supply response in the economy.

In practice, the distinction between stabilization and structural adjustment is often obscured by the fact that many of the same policy instruments, such as exchange rate devaluation and fiscal policy restraint are common to both areas. On the other hand, it is true that certain conflicts may arise between stabilization and structural adjustment, as illustrated by the fact that trade liberalization associated with structural adjustment may exacerbate the short-term macro-economic imbalances that stabilization programmes are designed to address. But, by and large, the numerous complementarities between stabilization and structural adjustment suggest a need to be aware of the broad differences between demand-contracting policies and those that are designed to restore balances through increased productivity and output.

The highly simplified diagram in Fig. 7.1 provides a framework that incorporates both the key elements of stabilization and structural adjustment, hereafter often referred to only as *adjustment*, or by the even more general term of *policy reform*. In any event, a few key elements of the links between adjustment and nutrition are elucidated in the framework. First, stabilization policies are largely imposed through limiting the public sector's role in the economy. More precisely, the impact of stabilization measures will be felt largely through reducing the level of government spending, and/or increasing revenues, which will subsequently affect public sector employment, household incomes, the nature and level of services and subsidies, and thereafter nutrition.

At the same time, structural adjustment policies will operate primarily through their effects on output. employment, factor payments, and prices. The concern here is that, in combination with efforts to stabilize the economy, expenditure-switching policies, such as exchange rate devaluation and trade liberalization, or institutional reforms that remove price controls and subsidies, may result in a variety of outcomes that threaten nutrition. These would be felt, for example, if net consumers

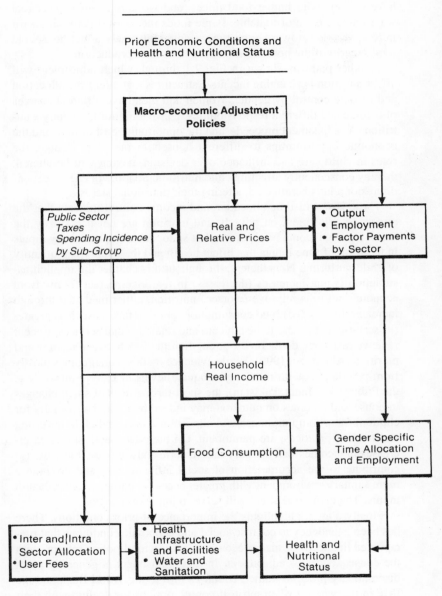

**Fig. 7.1** Policy reform and welfare outcomes

have to cope with higher food prices, and workers receive lower real wages as the price of tradable, staple foods increases. Likewise, a shift in relative prices toward export crops could adversely affect household food security if the poor are not engaged in their production.

Another pathway shown in Fig. 7.1 through which adjustment will affect nutrition is changing incentive structures that alter time allocation and income control by gender. Women and men have different sources of income and different responsibilities in providing for the family's nutrition. As adjustment proceeds, and the opportunity cost of time and the economic opportunities to different household members change, the roles in child care and influence over decision-making will be altered, thereby consequently affecting child nutrition. So too will energy expenditures of adults be affected, altering their nutritional status.

These issues of time allocation and income control indicate that the effects of adjustment on poverty and nutrition are not necessarily the same. Family income is important, but so too are complementary inputs in the form of time inputs that affect health and the quality and quantity of child nurturing. Nonetheless, throughout this chapter the implicit assumption is that increases (decreases) in real income that follow from economic reforms improve (worsen) nutrition, either mediated through increased (decreased) food consumption, or other factors such as greater (lesser) use and access to health care and related social services. Recent reviews cast some doubt on the strength of the link between income and nutrition (Alderman, 1990). While evidence on this matter comes mostly from populations with relatively adequate levels of calorie intake (e.g. the Philippines, India, Pakistan), the short-term effects of small changes in household incomes on nutrition may indeed be limited, especially for children for whom intrahousehold allocation issues, and child nurturing and feeding practices, are paramount. On the other hand, sustained increases in incomes will not only raise calorie consumption, but will also contribute to the accumulation of social infrastructure and promote a more sanitary environment with greater access to complementary health inputs. The combined effect will serve to improve nutrition.

Finally, Fig. 7.1 highlights the importance of prior conditions. There has been a tendency to confuse social and economic conditions that precipitated the need for macro-economic and sectoral policy reform, with the consequences of adjustment. In fact, adjustment is generally not a discretionary process. Rather, countries turn to the World Bank and the IMF in desperation when most, if not all, options for dealing with their acute economic crisis have been exhausted. These times of crisis, and the causes thereof, should not be viewed as the fault of reform, but as its challenge.

## PUBLIC EXPENDITURES

### Social Services

The state plays a potentially key role in terms of promoting development in general, and nutritional improvement in particular through public expenditure on health and related social services, such as education, as well as through subsidies on food. The two salient questions that arise in considering the impact of adjustment on nutrition, as mediated through fiscal policy, revolve around, first, how the level and nature of nutrition-related public expenditures change during adjustment and, second, the efficacy of monies that are spent.

The literature alleging harmful effects of adjustment on poverty focuses largely on the issue of reduced public spending, especially on social services. In fact, the experiences of middle-income countries in Latin America, as well as Asian nations, strongly suggest that adjustment involved fiscal contraction (Grosh, 1990; Pinstrup-Andersen, Jaramillo, and Stewart, 1987; Musgrove, 1987; Sahn, 1987). The question arises, however, as to whether that is relevant and representative of the process of reform in sub-Saharan Africa.

Recently-compiled evidence indicates no general pattern of declining total government expenditures in sub-Saharan Africa during the 1980s, the years when most countries were undergoing adjustment. Likewise, total expenditures as a share of GDP showed no secular trend, as the size of the state in the economy did not fall. One caveat to these findings, however, is that the interest payments as a share of total spending increased, implying a marginal decline in discretionary expenditures (Sahn, 1992).

Of greater relevance to the link with nutrition, however, is the intersectoral allocation of expenditures. The data from Africa also suggest no general pattern of decline in real health and education expenditures, those social services that are likely to have the most direct impact on nutrition during the period of adjustment. In addition, as shown in Fig. 7.2, the level of health and education expenditures as a percentage of GDP during the 1980s has been stable.

When these data are examined by country, it becomes apparent that there is no general pattern of change in terms of the share of government

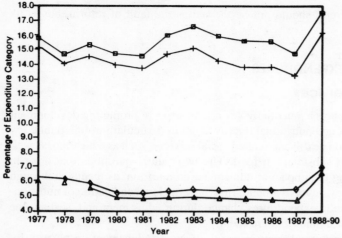

**Fig. 7.2** Health and Education Expenditures: percentage of total expenditures and total discretionary expenditures (i.e. net of interest)

Source: Sahn, 1992

**Notes:** Education data includes Botswana, Burkina Faso, Cameroon, Ethiopia, The Gambia, Ghana, Kenya, Lesotho, Liberia, Madagascar, Malawi, Mali, Mauritius, Niger, Nigeria, Sierra Leone, Swaziland, Togo, Uganda, Zambia, and Zimbabwe.

Health data includes Botswana, Burkina Faso, Cameroon, Ethiopia, Kenya, Liberia, Madagascar, Malawi, Mali, Mauritius, Niger, Nigeria, Rwanda, Swaziland, Toga, Uganda, Zambia, and Zimbabwe.

spending in the wake of the beginning of adjustment. Table 7.2 presents data on health and education spending in the period before and after the beginning of World Bank-sponsored adjustment programmes, both in terms of real health and education expenditures and health and education expenditures as a share of GDP. Once again, the evidence does not indicate any clear pattern of change subsequent to adjustment. What these data do show, however, is considerable variation from one country to the next. For example, while Ghana's real expenditure on health and education, and expenditures on health and education as a share of total expenditures, increased dramatically after adjustment, neighbouring Togo witnessed a decline, albeit of a much lower magnitude. Similarly, education expenditures fell markedly in Senegal, although those for health

**Table 7.2** Real education and health expenditures before/after adjustment (expressed in indices (1980=100)) and as a percentage of total discretionary government expenditures (i.e. net of interest)

| | Education Expenditures as percentage of total Discretionary Government Expenditure | | Real education expenditure expressed as indices (1980=100) | | Health Expenditures as percentage of total Discretionary Government Expenditure | | Real health expenditure expressed as indices (1980=100) | |
|---|---|---|---|---|---|---|---|---|
| | Before SAP | After SAP | Before SAP | After SAP | Before SAP | After SAP | Before SAP | After SAP |
| Burkina Faso | 19.2 | 16.7 | 119 | 134 | 6.4 | 5.5 | 105 | 118 |
| Cote d'Ivoire | 20.1 | 25.8 | 125 | 132 | 3.8 | 4.6 | 97 | 97 |
| The Gambia | 7.7 | 6.9 | 57 | 48 | – | – | | |
| Ghana | 20.5 | 23.0 | 58 | 99 | 7.1 | 9.8 | 67 | 132 |
| Kenya | 19.5 | 21.7 | 100 | 108 | 7.6 | 7.1 | 100 | 99 |
| Madagascar | 17.5 | 16.5 | 67 | 66 | 5.2 | 5.7 | 61 | 66 |
| Malawi | 11.4 | 15.6 | 112 | 124 | 5.6 | 7.8 | 97 | 100 |
| Mauritius | 17.6 | 17.0 | 99 | 95 | 7.8 | 8.8 | 101 | 115 |
| Niger | 14.2 | 14.0 | 63 | 70 | 4.2 | 4.8 | 84 | 106 |
| Nigeria | 9.4 | 7.4 | 94 | 49 | 2.5 | 2.4 | 81 | 48 |
| Senegal | 29.5 | 19.2 | 72 | 25 | 6.0 | 4.9 | 104 | 113 |
| Sierra Leone | 16.6 | 9.9 | 104 | 91 | 7.2 | 4.0 | – | – |
| Togo | 22.4 | 14.7 | 109 | 97 | 6.4 | 4.8 | – | – |
| Uganda | 13.1 | 13.3 | 103 | 191 | 5.0 | 3.7 | 113 | 155 |
| Zambia | 15.5 | 14.5 | 108 | 118 | 7.5 | 5.8 | 100 | 87 |
| Zimbabwe | 21.2 | 22.4 | 152 | 153 | 6.6 | 6.8 | 135 | 133 |

Source: Sahn, 1992

Notes: 'Before adjustment' is defined as the year in which the first Structural or Sectoral Adjustment Loan was signed with the World Bank, and the two previous years. 'After adjustment' is defined as the three years after the first adjustment loan was signed. If data were available for only one or two of the years in either period, their average value was used instead. Data from years prior to 1980 were not included for the real expenditure indices. For those countries whose loan agreements were signed in 1980 or 1981, such as Kenya, Malawi, and Mauritius, only data for 1980 and 1981 were included. If data were missing for one or more years, the average value was used for those years for which data were available.

were better protected. A final point is that the low index numbers for health and education for countries such as Madagascar, both before and after adjustment, show how, relative to 1980, real government spending fell dramatically during the crisis that preceded the beginning of the formal adjustment programme sponsored by the international financial institutions.

Formalizing much of this discussion using an econometric model, we obtain the elasticities of health and education expenditures in respect of

**Table 7.3** Elasticities of health and education expenditures with respect to total expenditures

| Elasticity with respect to total expenditures | Before adjustment | | After adjustment | |
|---|---|---|---|---|
| | Low-income countries | Middle-income countries | Low-income countries | Middle-ncome countries |
| Health | 0.63 | 0.83 | 0.93 | 1.13 |
| Education | 0.66 | 0.92 | 1.08 | 1.33 |

Source: Sahn, 1992

total expenditures and GDP, as shown in Table 7.3. First and foremost, the elasticities are higher after, rather than before, adjustment. This suggests that after adjustment began, social sector expenditures were more responsive to changes in total expenditures, increasing at a faster rate relative to total expenditures than was the case before adjustment. Second, the elasticities for education are somewhat higher than for health. Third, the elasticities are higher for middle-income than for low-income countries. So, for example, these numbers can be simply interpreted as a 10 per cent increase in total expenditures after adjustment led to a 9.3 per cent increase in health spending among low-income countries, and an 11.3 per cent increase in middle-income countries. The percentage change in response to a 10 per cent change in total expenditures during the pre-adjustment period was 6.6 and 9.2 for low- and middle-income countries, respectively.

The indication that adjustment has, in general, not reduced the financial commitment of the state to nutrition, as measured by state involvement in the delivery of social services, begs the critical issue: the effectiveness of social service expenditures in fostering improved nutrition. Though there are models that formally link social expenditures on the part of government to nutrition outcomes, we do know that it is not the aggregate sectoral expenditures but rather the intrasectoral allocation and the type and quality of services that are of paramount importance. On this count, the evidence is quite consistent: social sector services prior to adjustment were skewed toward the provision of secondary and university education, and health services were skewed toward secondary and tertiary health care.

Numerous illustrations of the bias in intrasectoral service delivery against the non-nutritionally vulnerable are extant. For example, only 6.8 per cent of Malawi's budget was spent on preventive services in

1987–88 (World Bank, 1988), and even in Tanzania, often cited as a model of social equity, only 5.9 per cent of the health budget was devoted to prevention, whereas more than two-thirds of the health budget was allocated to hospitals (World Bank, 1989). Similarly, primary health care in Ghana and Madagascar received only 20–25 per cent of the Ministry of Health budget during the 1980s, a figure that was only approximately 10 per cent in Cote d'Ivoire. In Kenya, during the latter half of the 1980s, the share of the total health expenditures allocated to preventive/promotive health care was between 3 and 5 per cent, and to rural health, between 9 and 15 per cent. The greater part of the budget was for hospitals and curative care. Similarly, only 12 per cent of the health budget in Zimbabwe was devoted to preventive care, whereas in Burundi the hospital sector absorbs 80 per cent of the recurrent budget in the health sector. In fact, of the countries for which data were available, the highest share of the recurrent budget allocated to primary health care was in Uganda, at 55 per cent (Sahn and Bernier, 1993).

While these country examples, by all indications representative of the general situation in Africa, highlight one aspect of the problem in the intrasectoral allocation of resources, in practice, there were other weaknesses in the budgeting process that transcended the discrimination against primary and preventive health care. The fact that wages and salaries had escalated to 90–95 per cent of the recurrent budget, at the expense of supplies, equipment, and pharmaceuticals, was further evidence of the misallocation of resources that contributed to the burgeoning crisis in the health delivery system.

In combination, the general pattern of health expenditures being biased toward curative health care—including acute care, laboratory services, and hospitalization, as well as protecting wages at the expense of supplies, equipment, and training—lowered the returns from government spending in terms of indicators of morbidity, mortality, and nutrition. This clearly argues for focusing adjustment on encouraging a shift in priorities in favour of preventive care, including targeted health services such as maternal and child care and immunizations, and other public health activities such as health education, communicable disease control, and environmental health measures. The question arises, therefore, whether there has been any reorientation of priorities during the adjustment period. In general, the analysis of expenditure patterns over time gives only little basis for encouragement. In most countries undertaking adjustment, such as Kenya, Madagascar, and Uganda, no shift in intrasectoral allocation is noted. Even more disturbing, in some countries, such as Cote d'Ivoire, the share of recurrent resources slotted for hospital care has actually increased during the period of adjustment. And, though there is limited evidence that some social sector adjustment programmes, such as in Ghana and Malawi, have been successful at reorienting social services toward the poor, such examples remain the exception, not the rule.

The slow pace and scarce examples of positive change in terms of restructuring the social sector is clearly a failure of policy. It reflects, first, that the early stages of reforms have been concentrated on macroeconomic stability, even in the area of fiscal policy. In more recent years, however, the concept of World Bank provision of social sector adjustment credits has emerged as an approach to donors leveraging policy changes in the social sectors with external finance. As a result, the focus on intrasectoral allocation of resources has been given more scrutiny. New pronouncements, and related programmes for reorienting health spending, have also emerged in Cote d'Ivoire, Kenya, Madagascar, and Zimbabwe, although, in most cases, it is too early to anticipate the results.

Second, the latitude for, and appropriateness of, donors to dictate how budgetary resources should be spent has severe limits. These limits are a function of practical considerations, such as that the depth of knowledge required to revamp the social sectors is beyond the attainment of external advices. Moreover, sovereignty of host governments over decision-making places additional limits of what can be imposed.

Nonetheless, in those few cases where it is possible to delineate how external financial flows and domestic revenue is spent, the evidence indicates that the former is more likely to be allocated to preventive and public health measures. For example, in Uganda, only 33 per cent of the government's own resources in the health sector were allocated to primary health care, in contrast to 83 per cent of the donor funds in 1988 and 1989. Indeed, since resources are fungible, it is impossible, in the absence of donor finance, to determine how the resources directly under the control of the government would have been allocated. Nonetheless, the figures suggest a difference in priority, and that external influence may in fact encourage a new set of allocative priorities.

In sum, the above discussion highlights a couple of important points. First, the quality and quantity of pre-adjustment public services were often dismal, reflecting the crisis in recurrent expenditures and rent-seeking that characterized African economies prior to reform. Second, although the evidence suggests that adjustment has not exacerbated this crisis in service delivery, whereby rationing of care is often biased against the nutritionally vulnerable in dire distress, there is little question that the restructuring required to make the social sectors effective and efficient will be costly and timely. Thus, additional human and financial resources, both part of and separate from adjustment operations, are required to address the limited quality and quantity of social sector services that were extant prior to adjustment. It is nonetheless important, in considering how to revitalize the social sector, not to lay general blame on the process of adjustment for the dismal condition of the health and education systems extant in African countries. Rather, it is better to recognize the scope for, and limitations of, the process of reform to ameliorate the deficiencies in social welfare programmes and infrastructure, so that complementary action may be taken, as discussed later in this chapter.

## Food Subsidies

The role of food subsidies in improving nutritional status is well documented, though these are often poorly targeted and incur substantial fiscal costs (Pinstrup-Andersen, 1988). However, most of the evidence on the nutritional impact of subsidies is from Asia and Latin America, with only a few studies conducted in Africa. This reflects a research bias since, in fact, most African countries were extensively engaged in food marketing and food-related income transfers.

As the process of economic adjustment often involves cancelling subsidies in response to unsustainable budget deficits, the question to be resolved is: what has been the nutritional impact of such reform measures? The answer is to be found in examining the beneficiaries of state intervention prior to adjustment. Specifically, the results of research from Africa present a picture, in contrast to that of Asia and of Latin America, where food subsidies were generally ineffective, and not just an inefficient means of transferring income to and protecting the nutritional status of poor. This reflected that subsidized goods were stringently rationed, generally limited to urban areas, and, even within urban areas, biased in favour of prosperous households that were effective rent-seekers.

More specifically, a number of studies point to this conclusion, the corollary of which is that reducing food subsidies will not have adverse effects on the vast majority of the nutritionally vulnerable. In Guinea, the government was engaged in supporting a dual-market structure, which made available subsidized food at as much as 70 per cent cheaper than the open market rate. However, access to such supplies was extremely limited. Only 5 per cent of the cereals purchased outside the capital were via the official market during the heyday of state controls in the mid-1980s. In the capital, Conakry, this figure was higher, reaching a peak of 25 per cent of cereal purchases. The evidence, however, is that access was skewed toward civil servants and professional workers, while the poor engaged in commercial activities: the informal sector, and service occupations received a considerably smaller amount of subsidized food, both in absolute and relative terms.

In Niger, the state-run subsidy was so ineffective as to preclude its demise having any adverse effect on the poor. In fact, access to low-priced commodities was limited primarily to institutional customers such as public enterprises and the army (Jabara, 1991). A similar situation was witnessed in Tanzania, where rationed food subsidies were limited largely to urban areas, and the poor were ineffective in capturing the associated rents (Sarris and van den Brink, 1993). Instead, the benefits accrued primarily to upper-income households (Amani et al., 1988). Mozambique is another country where the food subsidy was limited to major cities, Maputo and Beira. Furthermore, the households that were resident for a longer duration were more likely to have a ration card allowing access to subsidized commodities, while newly-arrived migrants, generally at greater nutritional risk, were less able to arrange for a ration card (Alderman, Sahn, and Arulpragasam, 1991). In combination with the fact that ration card-holders receive only a small share of the goods through official markets, the evidence clearly shows that access to subsidized food was discriminated against the poor; and among those needy households that did participate, the value of the subsidy was extremely limited as reliance on the open market remained high (Sahn and Desai, 1993).

There are other cases, for instance, in Madagascar and Zambia, where the subsidy did, in fact, provide an income transfer to most urban households, including those of the poor. In Madagascar, the adjustment programme involved withdrawal of the subsidy, which had deleterious consequences for the poor, whereas in Zambia, there was resistance to such reforms. However, the fact remains that in Madagascar, only an estimated 7 per cent of the country's poor reside in urban areas (Dorosh, Bernier, and Sarris, 1990). While there was undoubtedly a real income loss that contributed to nutritional stress among these poor urban households, the relatively small number of nutritionally vulnerable that suffered from the subsidy withdrawal suggests that this measure was sound economic policy. Such a policy change, however, should have been done in conjunction with designing a targeted compensatory mechanism for the poor, a subject that is discussed later in the chapter.

The general picture that emerges from these, and other, experiences is that withdrawal of subsidies has, in general, had marginal, if any, harmful effects on the nutritionally vulnerable. Not only were the subsidies strictly rationed, urban-based, and biased toward less needy households more proficient at rent-seeking, but, in addition, the vast majority of the poor were reliant on parallel free markets, where they made the most of their purchases. This suggests that the major mechanism through which prices, and hence nutrition, will be affected by adjustment revolves around the impact on open market prices instead of rationed subsidies. This issue will be further addressed in the next section.

## MARKET REFORMS

At the core of structural adjustment is the reduction of market distortions, so that prices more closely reflect their scarcity value. This is often achieved through exchange rate and trade policy reforms, as well as through liberalization of domestic marketing arrangements. These two sets of policies are complementary. The former is aimed at making prices of goods at the country's border more closely reflect those on international markets. Market liberalization is designed to lift restrictions that impede the transmission of market-determined prices to the consumer and producer. In combination, these policies are expected to affect prices paid by consumers, and earnings of farm and non-farm households. The issue of how structural adjustment affects open-market prices, and incomes, therefore requires attention.

### Food Prices

As intimated in the earlier discussion on food subsidies, the concern over reforming commercial policies on nutritional outcomes is the potential effect of escalating the prices for staple foods. This is expected since most staple grains are tradable goods, and one of the underlying purposes of adjustment is to raise the price of tradables relative to nontradables in order to improve the balance of payments situation (i.e. through encouraging exports and discouraging imports).

This theory does not, however, stand the test of practical experience.

The evidence from most (but not all) countries indicates that reform has *not* been accompanied by rising real market prices for food. This is once again explained by the characteristics of state intervention in economies prior to adjustment. To amplify, the underlying reason that adjustment policies, such as exchange rate devaluation, have generally not hiked up real market prices for staple goods is that the prices in open markets (as opposed to the rationed, subsidized prices) were already determined on the basis of the parallel exchange rate. That is, the grossly overvalued exchange rate, the correction of which has been the focus of adjustment policies, had become irrelevant for the vast majority of transactions that were occurring long before reform commenced. With the exception of the government, and those few privileged rent-seekers who exploited their connections with high-level government officials, traders and merchants were paying parallel market rates for foreign exchange to purchase the food destined for the open market. So when devaluation occurred, the parallel market price did not rise, neither for food nor for foreign exchange.

In fact, just the opposite occurred in a number of circumstances. Open-market food prices fell in countries such as Ghana (Alderman, 1990), Guinea, Somalia (Sahn and Alderman, 1987), and Tanzania (Sarris and van den Brink, 1993). The reasons generally revolved around a combination of two factors. First, the efficiency of markets improved as trading was officially sanctioned. Increased competition, and a reduction of the risk inherent in operating on parallel markets, even if implicitly sanctioned, contributed to lower prices.

Second, the infusion of foreign exchange through adjustment lending was directed largely toward consumables. That is, the foreign exchange that was auctioned, or made available through more liberalized regimes, often contributed to a sizeable increase in imports, much of which was food. But just as the process of liberalization, where it has occurred, has contributed to more efficient marketing, and lower costs to the consumers, it is also the case that where reforms have been slow in coming, the prices of staple grains on open markets remain artificially high. Two recent studies, one from Mozambique and the other from Zimbabwe, clearly illustrate this point.

In the case of Mozambique, traders were relegated to operating on 'illegal', although tolerated parallel markets, and could not import grain directly from inexpensive international suppliers. Instead, they either had to procure commodities from Swaziland and South Africa, paying high prices, owing to the risk premia and high transaction costs involved in such purchasing and dangerous overland transport; or they could illegally divert some of the sizeable amount of food aid that was supposedly destined for the official market. The consequence of engaging in either aspect of illegal trade was that merchants sold goods on the parallel market at prices that were in excess of world market prices plus a reasonable marketing margin. There was every reason to expect, however, that legalizing grain trade and cancelling the high transaction costs that existed would lower prices to the consumer (Alderman, Sahn, and Arulpragasam, 1991).

A similar situation was witnessed in Zimbabwe. The state control of grain markets exerted in the form of inter-regional trade restrictions and resale restrictions that block the sale of grain to low cost, informal sector millers and traders, resulted in long and circuitous marketing channels, and limited the availability of less expensive higher extraction maize meal that would appeal to the poor (Jayne *et al.*, 1991).

Yet another example of the same type of problem, namely, the reluctance to liberalize trade, and undertake needed economic adjustments, was found in the Sahel. According to Badiane (1989), persistent obstacles hindering crossborder and regional trade in foodgrains caused the consumer hardships. He pointed out that lifting trade restrictions would be especially useful for facilitating maize imports from the humid coast countries during the Sahel's periods of recurring droughts.

While these examples are not unusual, in many other cases such as The Gambia (Jabara, 1990), where the exchange rate devaluation and commercial policy reforms were implemented, no major changes in grain prices were noted. In fact, other than the instances where an explicit and effective subsidy was eliminated (as discussed for Madagascar and Zambia), evidence strongly supports that, for most countries, the exchange rate and market liberalization associated with adjustment has not had a deleterious effect on nutrition as mediated through prices. And in many cases, just the opposite effect was observed, as prices fell in the wake of liberalizing markets and fostering competition.

## Incomes and Producer Incentives

The changes in consumer prices discussed above constitute a key element in determining how incomes evolve during the process of adjustment, and in combination, the impact of food consumption and nutrition. In addressing the issue of the effects on nutrition as mediated through income and food consumption, we focus first on the rural areas, where the prevalence of malnutrition is considerably higher, as already discussed.

In order to gain a better understanding of the degree to which adjustment affects nutrition, through changes in incomes and prices, it is useful to examine the sources of income among the poor. Table 7.4 shows that agricultural income comprises between 39 and 76 per cent of the total, for a sample of diverse countries in which representative data were available. Of the agricultural income, production for home consumption is considerably more important than income generated from market sales. Furthermore, the income from marketing non-traded goods, whose price is not expected to be directly affected through adjustment, generally exceeds the income from sales of tradable foods and export crops (Table 7.5). This immediately suggests that even if policies such as exchange-rate devaluation brought about an increase in market prices for tradables as a consequence of adjustment, the short-term, first-round effects on the incomes of the poor will be small, albeit significant, in countries such as Cote d'Ivoire where export crops are an important component of the incomes of poor households.

When expenditure share data are examined for a number of countries, we find that the share of food expenditures derived from home consumption ranges from 32 per cent in The Gambia to 88 per cent in the west and south of Madagascar. In addition, in most cases market purchases are more likely to be for non-tradables than for tradable food products (Table 7.6). These data reinforce the message that the poor have considerable scope for buffering not only any decline in price incentives, but also any increase in retail prices.

A number of recent simulation models have taken this information on income and expenditure shares, and mapped the effects of observed adjustment-induced price changes, or the lack thereof, on smallholders' incomes during the 1980s. A study by Sahn and Sarris (1991) made the simplifying assumption of fixed shares in the consumption package and structure of agricultural production of low-income smallholders. The results, however, showed only minor changes in real incomes of the poor during adjustment in four countries. The reason for these small effects are threefold. First, actual changes in producer prices were less than anticipated, as many countries failed to eliminate the heavy taxation of smallholder export crops, despite it being an espoused objective of adjustment. Second, the pervasiveness of parallel markets before adjustment limited the magnitude of actual real price changes that occurred. A third factor in explaining the results was that the Sahn and Sarris model

**Table 7.4** Sources of per capita income of poor rural smallholder households, by country and region

| Income source | Ghana Forest | Ghana Sava-nnah | Tan-zania All | Cote d'Ivoire Forest | Cote d'Ivoire Sava-nnah | Malawi South | Madagascar Coast | Madagascar Plateau | The Gambia South | The Gambia Regio-nal | Kenya Regio-nal | Rwanda Regio-nal | Burkina Faso Sahe-lian | Burkina Faso Sudan-ian | Burkina Faso Guin-ean |
|---|---|---|---|---|---|---|---|---|---|---|---|---|---|---|---|
| **Shares** | | | | | | | | | | | | | | | |
| Agricultural income[a] | 0.57 | 0.68 | 0.73 | 0.76 | 0.81 | 0.51 | 0.42 | 0.39 | 0.48 | 0.57 | 0.54 | 0.45 | 0.49 | 0.59 | 0.56 |
| of which: | | | | | | | | | | | | | | | |
| Home consumption | 0.37 | 0.54 | 0.50 | 0.31 | 0.40 | 0.37 | 0.25 | 0.31 | 0.37 | 0.22 | 0.40 | 0.33 | – | – | – |
| Agricultural sales | 0.20 | 0.14 | 0.23 | 0.45 | 0.41 | 0.14 | 0.17 | 0.08 | 0.11 | 0.35 | 0.14 | 0.12 | – | – | – |
| Off-farm earned income[b] | 0.40 | 0.31 | 0.25 | 0.21 | 0.17 | 0.13 | 0.55 | 0.58 | 0.49 | 0.22 | 0.42 | 0.38 | 0.20 | 0.25 | 0.38 |
| Non-earned income[c] | 0.03 | 0.01 | 0.02 | 0.03 | 0.02 | 0.36 | 0.03 | 0.03 | 0.03 | 0.21 | 0.04 | 0.17 | 0.31 | 0.16 | 0.06 |
| Total | 1.00 | 1.00 | 1.00 | 1.00 | 1.00 | 1.00 | 1.00 | 1.00 | 1.00 | 1.00 | 1.00 | 1.00 | 1.00 | 1.00 | 1.00 |

Sources: Ghana, Tanzania, Cote d' Ivoire, Malawi, and Madagascar computed from sources mentioned in Sahn and Sarris (1991); The Gambia from Jabara *et al.*, (1991); Kenya, Rwanda, and Burkina Faso from von Braun and Pandya-Lorch (1991).

[a] Includes livestock.
[b] Includes wages, salaries, and own-account
[c] Includes income from transfers, remittances, and other non-earned sources

**Table 7.5** Agricultural income shares of rural smallholders

| Income source | Ghana Forest | Ghana Savannah | Tanzania All | Cote d'Ivoire Forest | Cote d'Ivoire Savannah | Malawi South | Madagascar Coast | Madagascar Plateau | Madagascar South | The Gambia Regional | Kenya Regional |
|---|---|---|---|---|---|---|---|---|---|---|---|
| Traded food[a] | 0.18 | 0.26 | 0.35 | 0.14 | 0.32 | 0.53 | 0.23 | 0.30 | 0.36 | 0.63 | 0.35 |
| Home consumed | 0.09 | 0.16 | 0.27 | 0.08 | 0.18 | 0.52 | 0.23 | 0.28 | 0.33 | 0.19 | – |
| sales | 0.09 | 0.10 | 0.09 | 0.06 | 0.14 | 0.01 | <0.01 | 0.02 | 0.03 | 0.44 | – |
| Non-traded food[b] | 0.70 | 0.73 | 0.61 | 0.41 | 0.46 | 0.24 | 0.46 | 0.69 | 0.58 | 0.37 | 0.45 |
| Home consumed | 0.57 | 0.63 | 0.42 | 0.32 | 0.31 | 0.20 | 0.35 | 0.51 | 0.44 | 0.20 | – |
| sales | 0.13 | 0.10 | 0.18 | 0.09 | 0.14 | 0.04 | 0.11 | 0.18 | 0.15 | 0.17 | – |
| Export crops[c] | 0.12 | 0.01 | 0.04 | 0.45 | 0.22 | 0.23 | 0.31 | 0.01 | 0.06 | 0.00 | 0.20 |
| Total | 1.00 | 1.00 | 1.00 | 1.00 | 1.00 | 1.00 | 1.00 | 1.00 | 1.00 | 1.00 | 1.00 |

Sources: Ghana, Tanzania, Cote d'Ivoire, Malawi, and Madagascar computed from sources mentioned in Sahn and Sarris (1991); The Gambia from Jabara et al., (1991); Kenya from IFPRI South Nyanza data set.

[a] Rice, maize, groundnuts, other traded food
[b] Millet, cassava, sweet potato, yams, other non-traded food
[c] Cocoa, tobacco, cotton, coffee, cola nuts, rubber, sugar, other exportables

**Table 7.6** Expenditure shares of rural smallholders

| Shares | Ghana | | Tanzania | Cote d'Ivoire | | Malawi | Madagascar | | | Gambia | Kenya | Cameroon |
| --- | --- | --- | --- | --- | --- | --- | --- | --- | --- | --- | --- | --- |
| | Forest | Savannah | All | Forest | Savannah | South | Coast | Plateau | South | Regional | Regional | National |
| Food share | 0.72 | 0.73 | 0.71 | 0.65 | 0.70 | 0.62 | 0.59 | 0.65 | 0.62 | 0.63 | 0.82 | 0.62 |
| of which: | | | | | | | | | | | | |
| Home consumption | 0.37 | 0.51 | 0.48 | 0.39 | 0.44 | 0.38 | 0.51 | 0.56 | 0.54 | 0.20 | 0.47 | 0.38 |
| Tradables | 0.06 | 0.10 | 0.18 | 0.08 | 0.15 | 0.27 | NA | NA | NA | 0.10 | NA | NA |
| Non-tradables | 0.31 | 0.41 | 0.30 | 0.31 | 0.29 | 0.11 | NA | NA | NA | 0.10 | NA | NA |
| Purchases | 0.35 | 0.22 | 0.23 | 0.26 | 0.26 | 0.24 | 0.08 | 0.09 | 0.07 | 0.43 | 0.35 | 0.24 |
| Tradables | 0.03 | 0.11 | 0.05 | 0.06 | 0.10 | 0.08 | NA | NA | NA | 0.24 | NA | NA |
| Non-tradables | 0.32 | 0.11 | 0.18 | 0.20 | 0.16 | 0.16 | NA | NA | NA | 0.19 | NA | NA |
| Non-food share | 0.28 | 0.27 | 0.29 | 0.35 | 0.30 | 0.38 | 0.41 | 0.35 | 0.38 | 0.37 | 0.18 | 0.38 |
| Total | 1.00 | 1.00 | 1.00 | 1.00 | 1.00 | 1.00 | 1.00 | 1.00 | 1.00 | 1.00 | 1.00 | 1.00 |

Sources: Ghana, Tanzania, Cote d'Ivoire, Malawi, Madagascar computed from sources mentioned in Sahn and Sarris (1991); The Gambia from Jabara *et al.* (1991); Cameroon computed from 1983-84 Household Budget Survey data tapes; Kenya from 1984-85 IFPRI South Nyanza data.

NA not available.

tends to underestimate potential gains from adjustment programmes that alter relative prices since the static simulation precludes switching crops and increasing output in response to price incentives.

Other recent work that examines the counterfactual with more sophisticated econometric and general equilibrium models shows that in countries such as Cameroon (Benjamin, 1993), Malawi (van Frausum and Sahn, 1993), Madagascar (Dorosh, 1992), Niger (Dorosh and Nssah, 1992), and Tanzania (Sarris and van den Brink, 1993), more aggressive pursuit of price and institutional reforms in export markets would have resulted in substantial increases in incomes to the rural poor. In all cases, the reluctance to undertake and the slow pace of marketing and/or exchange rate reform, both impeded recovery and had adverse distributional implications.

While a complete discussion on the income effects of adjustment in rural areas is beyond the scope of this chapter, and is reviewed elsewhere (Sahn, 1991), the preponderance of evidence leads to some general conclusions. First, the potential benefits from adjustment, especially during the early phases, were diminished by a reluctance to undertake true structural change on the part of policymakers. This reflected that pre-reform distortions often served the rent-seeking purposes of the elite and those involved in state-owned and state-operated enterprises. Second, the rural poor were rarely losers from reform, even in cases such as Cote d'Ivoire where stabilization brought a significant drop in GDP. This was largely due to their high degree of subsistence and their low reliance on the formal sector where most of the contraction occurred. Third, the most substantial gains for the rural poor accrued in those countries that seriously attempted to reduce the overt taxation of farmers and improve the rural–urban terms of trade. Fourth, where an attempt to truly liberalize markets and restore incentives was extant, such as in Ghana, Guinea, and Mozambique, institutional constraints often impeded a robust supply response in agriculture, slowing down the pace of improvements in incomes of rich and poor alike.

In respect of changes in urban incomes, the evidence suggests that, to the extent that real income declines followed from adjustment, they were concentrated largely in urban areas. Similarly, the greatest losers in urban areas were those who lost their jobs through reductions in the size of the civil service, as occurred in several countries. Urban incomes in countries such as Cameroon, in the wake of the decline in oil prices, and even neighboring Cote d'Ivoire with its large, well-paid, formal-sector labour force, both within and without government, were especially hard hit. However, mitigating the magnitude of the implications of job loss for those engaged in the civil service was a generous severance package such as that provided in Guinea and Ghana. In addition, prior to the retrenchment schemes, the value of real wages for public-sector workers had generally fallen dramatically. In particular, inflation from undisciplined fiscal and monetary policy dramatically eroded real formal-sector wages in the years prior to adjustment. As such, the data suggest that many public-sector workers were making a surprisingly small contribution to household incomes. Furthermore, moonlighting on the part of state workers, coupled with there being multiple income earners per household, reduced the negative shock of the contraction of the civil service in those few countries that have been serious about restructuring.

It is also noteworthy that, as part of restructuring of the civil service, adjustment programmes have dictated major increases in real wages for those who remain employed. The objective is simply to foster greater productivity through increasing the financial incentives to civil service workers. As such, countries as disparate as Guinea, Gambia, Ghana, and Mozambique have seen real civil service wages increase two or more times since the beginning of adjustment.

Of more critical importance than the plight of civil servants, who generally are not included among the most vulnerable, is that of the informal sector workers. Little empirical evidence exists on which to formulate any generalizations about the changes in their welfare since the beginning of adjustment. However, the indications of moderating urban food prices in many countries, and a boom in the availability of consumer goods and commercial activity in urban centres such as Accra, Conakry, Dar es Salaam, Maputo, and Mogadishu (before the dissolution of the adjustment programme and the civil war) would seem to suggest a burgeoning of informal sector activity and related small and micro-enterprises. There is, nonetheless, little question that these enterprises provided primarily low-paying jobs which were, for the most part, at best ensuring the minimum subsistence of the household. Clearly, the future challenge is to generate good-paying jobs, but to do so without relying on the state to maintain a bloated and unproductive civil service which, in many countries, ranging from Guinea to Niger to Madagascar, once guaranteed employment for all graduates, while in reality did little to protect the welfare of the poor.

## GENDER AND TIME USE

A key determinant of nutrition is the quality and quantity of time inputs into a variety of tasks, such as food preparation, breast-feeding, sanitation, and so forth. To the extent that adjustment affects the use of time, there will be an impact on nutrition. This is particularly important relative to a change in the incentive structure for market versus home production activities. Women first assume primary responsibility for child care, food preparation, and other home production activities, all of which may be diminished by greater participation in the labour market. Second, some studies suggest that there are higher costs of re-allocating time from direct (e.g. child care) to indirect (e.g. earning income) welfare, provisioning activities for women (Juster and Stafford, 1991). However, recent data from Guinea indicate that this generalization does not always hold, as leisure time for both men and women is high (Glick, Sahn, and Del Ninno, 1992). In the final analysis, however, without a full appreciation of the trade-offs between increased incomes and a reduction of time in home production, it is virtually impossible *a priori* to resolve the effects of such changes on the nutritional status of children and women.[1]

Another important gender-mediated effect of adjustment programmes on nutrition is the issue of income control.[2] Some research suggests that, along with increased incentives for cash-cropping, men will assume a more important role in earning income, and thus gain greater control over the allocation of income. Similarly, there is evidence, in some instances, that the preference ordering of men differs dramatically from that of women, with inputs into nutrition suffering when men assert greater control over the expenditure of income.

Countering these findings is other research that shows the resurgent role of women in trade and commerce as market liberalization proceeds, thereby putting income back into the hands of women, rather than of male-dominated parastatals. Similarly, there are mixed results of multivariate studies on proxies for income control on nutrition, such as the impact of the gender of the head of household.[3]

---

[1] For example, see Kennedy and Bouis (1989) where they show how regional resource endowments affect the manner in which changes in time use, commensurate with increased cash-cropping, had differential effects on nutrition.

[2] For a more detailed discussion of the issues relating to gender-specific income control, see Chapter 5: Collier (1990) and Elson (1990).

[3] It is important that any discussion of issues such as household headship be handled by using a multivariate approach, so as not to confuse association with causation.

While the gender-mediated impacts of adjustment on nutrition are a cause for concern, they suggest, first, that more empirical evidence needs to be brought to bear on these issues. These impacts are indeed complex, and have left recent reviews inconclusive (Sahn and Haddad, 1991; Haddad, 1991; MayaTech, 1991). Whether it be the fact that observed patterns of income earnings by individuals within the household are not exogenous, but interdependent, or the fact that there are complex patterns of bargaining that resolve the differences in the preference ordering of individual household members, there is a need for research to further explore these important processes.

Second, recognizing the potentially-harmful effects of adjustment as mediated through changes in gender roles and income controls is important in rousing awareness and encouraging vigilance to preclude such negative effects from materializing. In other words, it is crucial not to be blind to the role of gender in the allocation of household time and financial resources. At the same time, there is a need to be aware of the gender dimensions of the issue. This latter point cautions against impulsive assumption that deleterious nutritional consequences result from increased time inputs into income-earning activities by women; or, conversely, that child malnutrition will necessarily increase if men assume a larger role in income earning, such as when incentives for export-crop production increase and men are primarily engaged in such occupations. This need for caution suggests an urgency for more exhaustive research into the dynamics of time use and gender roles, and its relationship to adjustment.

## COMPENSATORY PROGRAMMES AND SOCIAL FUNDS

During the early part of the 1980s, structural adjustment was undertaken without serious consideration of the social consequences in general, and nutritional implications in specific. This situation changed markedly during the course of the decade. Undoubtedly, a significant contribution to the need to attend to the plight of the nutritionally vulnerable during the process of adjustment was attributable to the advocacy of UNICEF, as is embodied in the book *Adjustment with a Human Face*. Despite the fact that the causal link UNICEF made between adjustment and poverty was flawed, failing to recognize that the misguided policies which led to the economic crisis were the same as those that resulted in the stagnation and declining of living standards, the result of their arguments was to highlight the needs of the poor. This compelled action, particularly on

the part of the World Bank, to initiate and encourage special programmes to target services and incomes to the poor. A recent review of World
Bank programming by Alderman (1992) shows that since 1987 there has
been a marked increase in the likelihood that social-sector concerns be
explicitly integrated into adjustment lending in the form of various targeted interventions.

It is also the case that during the course of the decade there seems to
have been an evolution in terms of how nutrition and related programmes have been framed. Specifically, the early efforts to incorporate
nutrition objectives into adjustment lending were regarded as 'compensatory' programmes, designed to address the 'social costs' of adjustment.
This approach had some serious conceptual problems. First and foremost, the empirical basis for suggesting that the nutritionally vulnerable
were being harmed by adjustment was weak. Second, the clear losers in
adjustment programmes, at least in those countries that were serious
about making structural reforms (many of which were not, and therefore,
arguably should not be considered as having undergone structural adjustment) were groups such as civil servants and those with access to special
privileges and rationed services, such as free secondary education, hos-
pital-based care, and rationed food subsidies. These groups, for the most
part, were not the poor. Thus, there was a propensity for compensatory
programmes to incur the payment of high severance fees to retrenched
bureaucrats, providing special low-interest loans to former civil servants, completing unfinished housing projects for civil service workers,
and so forth.[4] While such initiatives may have considerable justification
for reasons of political economy, they are not to be confused with initiatives to reduce malnutrition.

These factors have led to a reframing of special and badly-needed
efforts to address the nutrition problems that exist in Africa among the
poor, those distressed by the economic policies that precipitated the need
for adjustment, and those that have failed to witness any appreciable
improvement in their standard of living since the slow and sometimes
lugubrious process of adjustment began. In particular, the concept of
special social funds or social action programmes to address poverty and
malnutrition has emerged, recognizing that there are comparatively few
new poor as a result of adjustment, despite that it is the challenge of

---

[4]Jolly and van der Hoeven (1989) report that the social programmes implemented most rapidly in Ghana were those directed to helping the civil servants, and the poor were not reached quickly or adequately.

reform to improve the plight of vulnerable groups. These funds, there-fore, take as their challenge addressing poverty and malnutrition, regard-less of its cause, without undercutting the fundamental tenets of economic reform (Alderman, 1992). Some of these funds are explicitly set up under the sponsorship of the World Bank, such as the Program to Mitigate the Social Costs of Adjustment (PAMSCAD) in Ghana,[5] while others, such as the social plan in Tanzania which receives a portion of its funding from the World Bank, are not explicitly part of the adjustment process.

Regardless of whether viewed as compensation for adjustment, or more accurately as efforts to rectify social ills in the short term in recog-nition of the limitations of adjustment, social funds do provide quick dispersing resources which can be utilized in an innovative fashion to reduce poverty and malnutrition. As social funds become of increasing importance in Africa, however, a range of problems has emerged in translating the theory of social action into effective projects. First, the data required for targeting programmes in Africa are not readily avail-able. For example, when PAMSCAD was putting together its portfolio of social projects, it did so in an information vacuum which was sub-sequently filled by the Ghana Living Standards Survey. Nonetheless, the imperative of doing something, quickly, precluded waiting for what was to prove extremely valuable household data on the causes, charac-teristics, and prevalence of poverty. While this problem of policymaking and programme design in the absence of adequate information is not new, it is particularly problematic in the context of targeted interven-tions.[6]

Second, the technical and managerial capabilities for selecting the appropriate forms of intervention, and managing the programmes, is often conspicuous by its absence. This suggests that there is a need to

---

[5]PAMSCAD was one of the forerunners of the concept of special action to ame-liorate malnutrition in conjunction with adjustment. It was framed in terms of compensating for adjustment rather than addressing the chronic malnutrition that was extant prior to the beginning of reform. Being a member of the initial World Bank mission to set up PAMSCAD, this misrepresentation of the cause of the problem was recognized at the earliest stages. However, we felt that touting the negative effects of adjustment was an effective impetus in generating financial support from the donors for the social programmes.

[6]Van der Hoeven (1991) argues that the concept of quick-disbursing social funds aimed at comprehensively addressing the poverty problem was ill-conceived and overtly optimistic.

start with small, pilot schemes. The limited coverage of such small-scale initiatives, however, often fails to correspond to other social and political imperatives of doing something big, quickly.

A third and related point concerns the concept of relying on non-governmental organizations (NGOs) to implement the social funds. Certainly, searching for community-based alternatives to the central control of the state has considerable merit, especially in much of Africa where the urban elite, who hold the reigns of power and control the treasury, have shown a lack of concern at best, and disdain at worst, for the peasantry and informal sector. However, the capacity and experience of NGOs in Africa is generally quite limited, particularly with regard to organizing large-scale interventions. Furthermore, in practice, NGOs often are, or simply become, extensions of the state and, in essence, quasi-state institutions, especially when large sums of money are perceived to be available to such civil institutions. In addition, the focus on NGOs is potentially counter to the objective of the SALs, namely, to strengthen and build up government's capacity for delivering social services equitably and efficiently.[7]

Fourth, social funds are, in theory, finance that is additional to normal aid flows. They are thus dependent on special financing from the donors. The pace of gaining financial commitments, and the subsequent disbursement of the funds realized, has been slow in many cases, impeding implementation of planned action.

Despite these concerns, to the extent that the process of adjustment provides increased impetus for addressing the acute social problems in Africa, social funds are indeed a potentially useful instrument for reducing malnutrition. However, it is probably counterproductive to have unrealistic expectations about the pace at which these efforts can be organized, especially given the limitations of data, management, and planning capacity, and related institutional constraints on the part of donors.

## CONCLUSIONS

This review has suggested that the evidence on the nutritional impact of

---

[7] In combination, these questions about whether and to what extent compensatory programmes should fall outside normal, state, bureaucratic channels was reported to be one of the reasons for the delay in the implementation of PAM-SCAD in Ghana (van der Hoeven, 1991).

adjustment programmes is mixed, generally not indicating any major deleterious effects, but producing meager evidence that many of the underlying causes of malnutrition have been ameliorated. Those countries where the effects of adjustment have been most harsh, such as Zaire, Somalia, and Zambia, are precisely the ones that have been least committed to the process. Instead, all the structural features that contributed to widespread poverty and malnutrition remain in those instances where the process of adjustment was at best sporadic and ineffectual in bringing about change. In contrast, improvements in incomes, and investments in social and physical infrastructure, and human capital, which are the basis for reducing malnutrition, have tended to occur in countries that have been committed to meaningful policy reform such as Ghana, Guinea, and, more recently, Madagascar and Tanzania.

It is also the case that certain groups of urban households, particularly those who lost their formal sector jobs as civil servants or in heavily subsidized public enterprises, have undoubtedly witnessed a decline in real incomes. This is especially so in countries where the process of stabilization has dominated over structural reforms, such as when the oil boom ended in Cameroon, or the unsustainable investment boom collapsed in Cote d'Ivoire. But, with few exceptions, the situation for the urban poor primarily engaged in the informal sector has likely not worsened, and in many cases has improved marginally with the increase in commercial activities and the availability of consumer goods.

Similarly, small holders in rural areas have perhaps witnessed marginal improvements in their incomes and living standards commensurate with a shift in the urban–rural terms of trade toward rural areas. This may have had some positive effect on household calorie intake and nutrition. However, there is little solid empirical evidence one way or the other to suggest that these changes in incomes were large enough to bring about improvement in the stock of knowledge and public and private investments in social infrastructure that will contribute to less chronic and acute malnutrition.

In terms of the role of the state in directly providing subsidies, prior to adjustment, rural areas were poorly served by urban-based health and social services, and benefited little from the subsidies on food and other goods that accrued primarily to the elite. Thus, even if cutbacks in the social sectors had occurred, which, by and large, they did not, such contractionary measures would have had limited deleterious effects because of the skewed nature of spending in favour of hospitals and curative care. The more salient question, therefore, is whether adjustment has brought about a reallocation of resources toward providing services that are targeted to the needs of the poor; the answer, unfortunately, has, for the most part, been 'no'.

There is scattered evidence to suggest that adjustment has, in some cases, raised the level of work of women outside the home, or altered income control with its potential deleterious impact on nutrition. However, the complex processes that determine the earnings of different family members, how time allocation affects nutrition and commodity demands, and the bargaining processes that determine intrahousehold allocation preclude arriving at simple and categorical statements as to the gender-mediated effects of adjustment on nutritional status (Stewart, 1991a; Haddad, 1991).

While most of the early criticism that implied that adjustment had deleterious impacts on nutrition is thus not substantiated, and if anything the direction of change has likely been positive, the fact is that the call for a human face to adjustment help put malnutrition, regardless of its cause, where it belongs at the centre of the debate on how to promote economic development. The growth of social funds and action programmes, as well as the discussion of poverty issues within World Bank adjustment loan documents, is testament to the partial success of this strategy, a change that has been documented by those within the World Bank (Ribe and Carvalho, 1990; Alderman, 1992), as well as those on the outside (Stewart, 1991b).

Likewise, there is a growing acceptance that nutritional concerns are compatible with structural reforms which address the distortions and failures of the developmental state, and the abuse of influence that translated into excessive rent-seeking and inefficiencies. While the extent to which the predatory actions of the state prior to adjustment has been reversed varies dramatically from one country to the other, there is a growing acceptance that nutrition was hampered by the conditions prior to adjustment. Similarly, the fact that state disengagement alone is not the answer to the need for restoring growth or eliminating malnutrition is a message that is becoming increasingly acknowledged. State investment in physical and social welfare, with the recognition that human capital development will bring about substantial, if not more difficult, to measure returns, is a key component of any growth strategy. But those investments, both in terms of programmes and infrastructure, need to be designed to encourage complementary investments by the private sector, and community-based action to improve and protect human resources. This challenge to the state is one of reorienting its role away from the allocation of privileges, as well as the production of goods and services, to that of setting the correct legal, regulatory, and incentive framework, generating requisite information and technology, and building institutional capacity in state and civil institutions for providing the requisite know-how in, for example, the design of appropriate nutrition interventions based on appropriate information. This is indeed an ambitious agenda, but one that is key to the success of adjustment in Africa, in both broad economic and more narrow nutritional terms.

## REFERENCES

Alderman, Harold (1992). Nutritional considerations in bank lending for economic adjustment. Paper prepared for the 12th Agricultural Symposium, World Bank, 8–10 January 1992.

Alderman, Harold (1990). Nutritional status in Ghana and its determinants. Cornell Food and Nutrition Policy Program Working Paper No. 1, Cornell University, Ithaca, New York.

Alderman, Harold, Sahn, David E., and Arulpragasam, Jehan (1991). Food subsidies in an environment of distorted exchange rates: Evidence from Mozambique. *Food Policy,* 395–404.

Amani, H. K. R., *et al.* (1988). Effects of market liberalization on food security in Tanzania. In: Rukuni, M. and Bernstein, R. (eds). *Southern Africa: Food Security Policy Options.* Proceedings of the 3rd Annual Conference on Food Security Research in Southern Africa, 1–5 November 1987. Harare: Department of Agricultural Economics and Extension, University of Zimbabwe/Michigan State University Food Security Research Project.

Badiane, O. (1989). The potential for an Espace Regional Cerealier (ERC) Ithaca, among West African countries and its possible contribution to food security. Paper presented at the Seminar on Regional Cereals Markets in West Africa, Lome, CILSS/OECD/Club du Sahel.

Benjamin, Nancy (1993). Income distribution and adjustment in an agricultural economy: A general equilibrium analysis of Cameroon. Cornell Food and Nutrition Policy Program Working Paper, Cornell University, Ithaca, New York.

Collier, P. (1991). Gender aspects of labour allocation during structural adjustment. Unit for the Study of Africa Economies, Oxford University, Oxford.

Cornia, Giovanni A., Jolly, Richard, and Stewart, Frances (eds). (1987). *Adjustment with a Human Face: Protecting the Vulnerable and Promoting Growth.* A Study by UNICEF, Clarendon Press, Oxford.

Demographic and Health Surveys (DHS) (1989). *Uganda: Demographic and Health Survey 1988/1989.* Institute for Resource Development/Westinghouse, Columbia, MD.

Dorosh, Paul A. (1992). A computable general equilibrium model for Madagascar: Equations and parameters. Cornell Food and Nutrition Policy Program, Washington, D.C.

Dorosh, Paul A. and Nssah, B. Essama (1992). External shocks, policy reform and income distribution in Niger. Cornell Food and Nutrition Policy Program, Washington, D.C.

Dorosh, Paul A., Bernier, Rene E., and Sarris, Alexander H. (1990). *Macroeconomic Adjustment and the Poor: The Case of Madagascar.* Cornell Food and Nutrition Policy Program Monograph No. 9. Cornell University, Ithaca, New York.

Elson, D. (1991). Gender and adjustment in the 1990s: An update on evidence and strategies. Economics Department, University of Manchester, Manchester.

Glick, Peter, Sahn, David E., and del Ninno, Carlo (1992). Labour markets and time allocation in Conakry. Cornell Food and Nutrition Policy Program Bulletin No. 6. Cornell University, Ithaca, New York.

Grosh, Margaret E. (1990). Social spending in Latin America: The story of the 1980s. World Bank Discussion Paper No. 106. World Bank, Washington, D.C.

Haddad, Lawrence (1991). Gender and adjustment: Theory and evidence to date. Paper presented at the Workshop on the Effects of Policies and Programmes on Women, 16 January 1992, International Policy Research Institute, Washington, D.C.

Jabara, Cathy L. (1991). *Structural Adjustment and Stabilization in Niger: Macro-economic Consequences and Impacts on the Poor.* Cornell Food and Nutrition Policy Program Monograph No. 11. Cornell University, Ithaca, New York.

Jabara, Cathy L. (1990). *Economic Reform and Poverty in The Gambia: A Survey of Pre- and Post-ERP Experience.* Cornell Food and Nutrition Policy Program Monograph No. 8. Cornell University, Ithaca, New York.

Jabara, Cathy L., Tolvanen, Marjatta, Lundberg, Mattias K. A., and Wadda, Rohey. *Incomes, Nutrition, and Poverty in The Gambia: Results from the CFNPP Household Survey.* Cornell Food and Nutrition Policy Program, Cornell University, Ithaca, New York.

Jayne, T. S., Rukuni, M., Hajek, M., Sithole, G., and Mudinu, G. (1991). *Structural Adjustment and Food Security in Zimbabwe: Strategies to Maintain Access to Maize by Low-Income Groups during Maize Market Restructuring.* University of Zambia, Harare and Michigan State University.

Jolly, R. and van der Hoeven, R. (1989). Protecting the poor and vulnerable during adjustment: The case of Ghana. Mimeo, UNICEF, New York.

Juster, F. T. and Stafford, F. P. (1991). The allocation of time: Empirical findings, behavioural models, and problems of measurements. *Journal of Economic Literature.* XXIX (June).

Kennedy, E. and Bouis, H. (1989). *Traditional Cash Crop Schemes Effects on Production, Consumption, and Nutrition: Sugarcane in the Philippines and Kenya.* International Food Policy Research Institute, Washington, D.C.

MayaTech (1991). *Gender and Adjustment.* Series TR 91–1026–02. The MayaTech Corporation, Silver Spring, MD.

Musgrove, P. (1987). The economic crisis and its impact on health and health care in Latin America and the Caribbean. *International Journal of Health Services,* 17(3), 411–41.

Pinstrup-Andersen, Per (ed). (1988). *Food Subsidies in Developing Countries.* The Johns Hopkins University Press in cooperation with the International Food Policy Research Institute, Baltimore, MD.

Pinstrup-Andersen, P., Jaramillo, M., and Stewart, F. (1987). The impact on current expenditure. In: Jolly, R. (ed). *Adjustment with a Human Face*. Clarendon Press, Oxford.

Ribe, Helena and Carvalho, Soniya (1990). World Bank treatment of the social impact of adjustment programmes. World Bank PRE Working Paper 521, World Bank, Washington, D.C.

Sahn, David E. and Bernier, Rene (1993). *Evidence from Africa on the International allocation of social sector expenditures*. Cornell Food and Nutrition Policy Program Working Paper No. 45, Cornell University, Ithaca, New York.

Sahn, David E. (1992). Public expenditures in sub-Saharan Africa during a period of economic reforms. *World Development*.

Sahn, David E. (1991). Has policy reform hurt the poor in Africa? Prepared for the World Bank Meeting of the Special Program of Assistance, Tokyo, October 1991.

Sahn, David E. (1987). Changes in the living standards of the poor in Sri Lanka during a period of macroeconomic restructuring. *World Development*, **15**(6).

Sahn, David E. and Desai, J. (1993). *The emergence of parallel market in a transition economy: The case of Mozambique*. Cornell Food and Nutrition Policy Program Working Paper. Cornell University, Ithaca, New York.

Sahn, David E. and Alderman, Harold (1987). The role of the foreign exchange and commodity auctions in trade, agriculture, and consumption in Somalia. International Food Policy Research Institute, Washington, D.C.

Sahn, David E. and Haddad, Lawrence (1991). The gender; impacts of structural adjustment programmes in Africa: Discussion. *American Journal of Agricultural Economics*, December.

Sahn, David E. and Sarris, Alexander H. (1991). Structural adjustment and rural smallholder welfare: A comparative analysis. *World Bank Economic Review*, June.

Sarris, Alexander H. and van den Brink, Rogier (1993). *Economic Policy and Household Welfare during Crisis and Adjustment in Tanzania*. New York University Press, New York.

Stewart, F. (1991a). The many faces of adjustment. *World Development*, **19**(12), 1847–64.

Stewart, F. (1991b). Protecting the poor during adjustment in Latin America and the Caribbean in the 1980s: How adequate was the World Bank response? Paper presented for Cornell Working on Macroeconomic Crises, Policy Reform and the Poor in Latin America, CIAT, Cali, Columbia, 1–4 October 1991.

van der Hoeven, R. (1991). Adjustment with a human face: Still relevant or overtaken by events? *World Development*, **19**(12), 1835–46.

van Frausum, Yves and Sahn, David E. (1993). An econometric model for Malawi: Measuring the effects of external shocks and policies. *Journal of Policy Modeling*.

von Braun, Joachim and Lorch, Rajul Pandya (eds). (1991). Income sources of malnourished people in rural areas: Microlevel information and policy implications. Working Paper on Commercialization of Agriculture and Nutrition No. 5, International Food Policy Research Institute, Washington, D.C.

World Bank (1989). *Tanzania: Public Expenditure Review*. World Bank, Washington, D.C.

World Bank (1988). *Malawi: Public Expenditure Review*. World Bank, Washington, D.C.

# 8

# Nutritional Status in Egypt: A Case Study

## MOHAMED AMR HUSSEIN AND WAFAA A. MOUSSA

## INTRODUCTION

Nutrition is one of the most important factors influencing the quality of human life in a major part of the world. While over-nutrition is sometimes a problem, undernutrition is chiefly responsible for the high rate of infant and young child mortality. In those who survive, it retards growth and development and lowers resistance to infections and environmental hazards. Maternal malnutrition is widespread, ruining the health of women and their infants. Subclinical malnutrition in adults reduces their work capacity, thereby disrupting socio-economic development. Malnutrition, therefore, is not merely a constant handicap to public health in the world today, but is also both a result and a cause of social and economic underdevelopment.

The importance of the role of nutrition in development programmes was realized in Egypt during the 1940s when nutrition activities were initiated. In the late 1940s, the nutrition corps in the Ministry of Health was established and formed the nucleus of the Nutrition Institute (NI) which was fully developed in 1955 as Egypt's main official body for nutrition care.

## NUTRITION AND DIET-RELATED PROBLEMS: NATURE AND DIMENSION

Protein–energy malnutrition (PEM) and iron deficiency anaemia were identified as the most prevalent types of malnutrition in Egypt. This has been revealed through several nutritional status surveys of different sectors of the population in diverse geographic areas (urban and rural) conducted by the NI as well as other research institutions. In many of these surveys, determinants of health and nutritional status—mainly food consumption, feeding and weaning practices, prevalence of infection, as well as socio-cultural and other ecological factors—have been studied. The relationships between PEM and all these factors were consolidated. Pre-schoolers, under the age of six years, are considered the most vulnerable group, and their nutritional status is accepted as a sensitive indicator of the nutritional status of the whole community. Data presented on this topic are compiled from only community-based national studies, mainly the ARE Nutritional Status Survey (NSS) 1978, the National Food Consumption Study (NI, Aly *et al.*, 1981), the Health Profile of Egypt (HPE), and the Health Examination Survey (HES) conducted by the Ministry of Health (MOH) in 1984 (Moussa, 1988). An update on a 10 per cent sub-sample of the ARE Nutritional Status Survey was conducted by NI in 1986 (Hussein *et al.*, 1989).

## Protein–Energy Malnutrition (PEM) and Chronic Dietary Energy Deficiency

The first National Nutrition Status Survey (1978) revealed that the prevalence of undernutrition, whether wasting or stunting, among pre-schoolers was more pronounced in rural than urban areas. The under-privileged districts of Cairo and Giza were more seriously affected than other urban areas. However, for Cairo as a whole, the proportion of normal pre-schoolers registered the highest, as concluded by the HPE–HES survey. Infants and children in the age group 6–23 months were the most severely exposed to acute undernutrition or wasting, while the 12–35 month age group showed the highest prevalence of chronic undernutrition or stunting. For the entire representative sample of Egypt (6–71 months age group), the total undernutrition or PEM, as measured by the weight-for-age per cent of the reference median (<90 per cent WHO/NCHS standards), was prevalent among 46.8 per cent. Wasting, denoting current acute undernutrition indicated by weight-for-height less than 80 per cent, was prevalent among only 1.3 per cent of the sample. Stunting, denoting chronic undernutrition (height-for-age less than 90 per cent) covered 21.2 per cent of the sample. However, among the special elite group this rate was only 1.1 per cent, which proves that growth retardation is mainly an environmental problem.

Table 8.1 Per cent distribution of pre-school children below cut-off levels for various anthropometric indices by age, Egypt 1978 and 1986 (34 sites)

| Age | Acute undernutrition — Weight-for-height per cent of median | | | | Chronic undernutrition — Height-for-age per cent of median | | | | Waterlow classification | | | | | | Gomez (weight-for-age) | | | | | |
|---|---|---|---|---|---|---|---|---|---|---|---|---|---|---|---|---|---|---|---|---|
| | Severe <80.0 | | Moderate 80.0–84.9 | | Severe <85.0 | | Moderate 85.0–89.9 | | Wasting and stunting <80Wt/Ht <90+Ht/Age | | Wasting <80 Wt/Ht 90+Wt/Ht | | Stunting <90 Ht/Age 80+Wt/Ht | | 3rd degree <60 | | 2nd degree 60–74.9 | | 1st degree 75–89.9 | |
| 6–11 | 3.3 | 9.0 | — | 6.3 | 3.3 | 2.7 | 6.7 | 16.2 | 1.1 | 8.2 | 7.8 | 18.2 | 2.2 | 0.9 | 3.3 | 4.5 | 8.9 | 12.6 | 44.4 | 29.7 |
| 12–23 | 2.0 | 6.4 | 4.9 | 6.8 | 8.5 | 14.1 | 22.8 | 23.2 | 1.6 | 3.2 | 30.9 | 34.2 | 0.4 | 3.2 | 2.8 | 5.4 | 21.1 | 18.6 | 51.2 | 43.4 |
| 24–35 | 0.5 | 2.4 | 2.5 | 4.9 | 9.3 | 5.9 | 23.2 | 18.5 | — | 1.9 | 32.0 | 23.9 | 0.5 | 0.5 | 1.5 | — | 9.8 | 9.8 | 38.2 | 43.7 |
| 36–47 | — | 1.6 | 0.5 | — | 6.5 | 4.7 | 18.4 | 19.5 | — | 1.1 | 24.9 | 22.9 | — | 0.5 | — | 1.1 | 3.2 | 4.2 | 33.9 | 33.7 |
| 48–59 | 0.7 | — | — | 0.7 | 6.7 | 5.9 | 20.7 | 11.8 | 0.7 | — | 27.4 | 17.0 | — | — | 0.7 | 0.7 | 5.9 | 2.2 | 35.6 | 35.3 |
| 60–71 | 2.3 | 2.8 | — | 1.4 | 4.5 | 3.4 | 18.2 | 13.8 | 1.5 | 2.1 | 22.0 | 16.5 | 0.8 | 0.7 | 1.5 | 1.4 | 6.1 | 6.2 | 35.6 | 30.1 |
| Total | 1.3 | 3.6 | 1.8 | 3.5 | 7.1 | 6.8 | 19.8 | 17.9 | 0.8 | 2.4 | 26.2 | 23.4 | 0.5 | 1.1 | 1.6 | 2.2 | 10.3 | 9.4 | 40.5 | 35.8 |

Hussein, M. A., Hassan, H. A., Noor, E. F., and El-Shafie, M. (1989). Nutritional assessment of pre-school children in Egypt, *Gza. Egypt. Paed. Ass.*, **37** (1–2).

A comparison of the results of the HPE–HES survey, conducted almost 5–6 years after the ARE–NSS (1978), showing the current trends in nutritional status, revealed increase in all forms of PEM (mild, moderate, and severe), from 46.8 per cent to 51.9 per cent. These results were also confirmed by the 1986 Nutritional Status Survey (NSS) update (Table 8.1). Due to the successful national programme of diarrhoeal disease control, victims of severe dehydration, who would otherwise have succumbed, have survived, but the proportion of severely malnourished children has increased.

In spite of the apparent improvement in Egypt's socio-economic status, there is no parallel transformation in the nutritional status during almost a decade. This may be due to the considerable rise in consumer food prices, as will be discussed later. A study of weights and heights, from the first year till 70 years and above, of a representative sample of Egyptians (HPE–HES–Moussa, 1989), as well as school children in Cairo and other governorates (Abdou and Mahfouz, 1968; Aly et al., 1975), revealed that height is more retarded than weight as compared with the international reference standards (WHO/NCHS), both in the pre-school and school age groups (<18 years) (Fig. 8.1a and b). Growth retardation, which is manifest from 6 months of age, is perceptibly worse at the end of the first year and is not corrected till adulthood.

Weights of adults aged 20–70 years and above in urban areas show a tendency to overweight, and even obesity, in the age group 30 to 60 years, particularly in the case of females. The mean height of men and women from 20-, 30-, 40-, 50-, and 70+ registers a decrease with age. This may denote that the heights of male and female populations of recent generations are improving in comparison with those of former generations. This phenomenon conforms with the general improvement in socio-economic standards.

## MICRONUTRIENT DEFICIENCIES

### Iron Deficiency Anaemia

*Prevalence among pre-school age children*

According to WHO (1968, 1990), a child from the age of 6 months to 6 years is considered anaemic if his haemoglobin concentration is less than 11 g per 100 ml blood. Results of the ARE–NSS (1978) revealed that 38 per cent of the total sample of pre-school children were anaemic. The prevalence of anaemia was the lowest among the special elite group

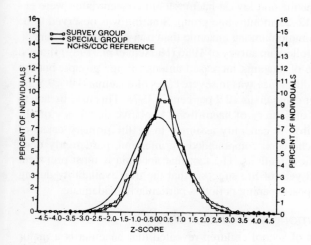

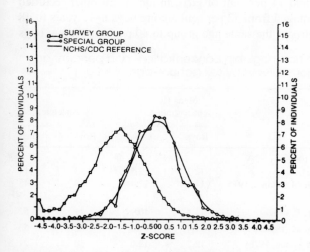

**Fig. 8.1 (a)** Egypt National Nutrition Assessment Survey, 1978 weight-for-height Z-score distribution

**Fig. 8.1 (b)** Egypt National Nutrition Assessment Survey, 1978 height-for-age Z-score distribution

(16.9 per cent), and the highest in rural areas (44 per cent). The highest prevalence of anaemia and lowest haemoglobin concentration were encountered in the 12–23 months age group. Stunting was observed to be nearly twice as common among anaemic than non-anaemic children.

Results of the follow up survey of 1986 (Hussein *et al.*, 1989) showed that the incidence of anaemia increased among all age groups, but the most remarkable difference was in severe cases of anaemia (Hb <9.5 gm per cent): 26.8 per cent versus 12.2 per cent in 1978. This may be due to the rise in prices of sources of haem iron. A relative deficiency of absorbable dietary iron is generally assumed to be the primary cause of anaemia in pre-schoolers, compounded by infection, particularly diarrhoea and parasitic infections. The fact that anaemia is most prevalent during the second year of life suggests that the iron availability during the weaning and post-weaning period is particularly inadequate.

## Prevalence among school age children

Scattered surveys of school children revealed that anaemia is a major nutritional problem among this age group (Table 8.2). Apart from a 1962 survey conducted in Cairo where anaemia was prevalent only among 13 per cent of boys and 11 per cent of girls, in almost all other recorded surveys anaemia ranged from 52 per cent among boys 6–12 years to 48 per cent among girls of the same age group to 40 per cent among boys

**Table 8.2** Mean haemoglobin concentrations and per cent anaemics in various surveys by sex (school–age children)

| Survey | Mean Hb concentration | | % Anaemic | |
|---|---|---|---|---|
| | Boys | Girls | Boys | Girls |
| Cairo school children 1962 (Abdou *et al.*, 1967c) | 12.7 | 12.5 | 13 | 11 |
| Follow up of Cairo school children, 1975 (Said *et al.*, 1980) | 11.6 | 11.4 | 39 | 45 |
| Asyut 1962 (Abdou *et al.*, 1967b) | 11.1 | 10.9 | 41 | 52 |
| Aswan 1962 (Abdou *et al.*, 1967b) | 11.4 | 11.0 | 53 | 56 |
| Aswan 1971 (Said and Abdou, 1978) | 12.2 | 12.6 | 30 | 21 |
| Beheira 1965–66 (Abdou *et al.*, 1968b) | | | | |
|     6–12 years | 11.2 | 11.2 | 52 | 48 |
|     12–18 years | 11.6 | 11.4 | 40 | 45 |
| HES–HPE     6–12 years (Moussa, 1988) | — | — | 44.7 | 45.2 |

of 12–18 years and 45 per cent among girls of the same age group. Anaemia was higher in males in the 6–12 year age group, but higher in females aged 12–18 years mostly due to difference in exposure to parasites and physiological causes (Abdou *et al.*, 1967b; Aly *et al.*, 1980; Moussa, 1988a).

The only national study in which haemoglobin (Hb) concentration using WHO levels was determined for children in the age group 6–12 years was the HPE–HES during 1983–84, reported by Moussa (1988). Anaemia was observed among 44.7 per cent of the boys and 45.2 per cent of the girls. It was more common among obese school-age children than among those suffering from severe undernutrition. Anaemia was much less prevalent in Cairo than in other areas.

## Prevalence among mothers

Haemoglobin data on mothers of children examined during the ARE National Nutrition Survey (NI/CDC, 1978) are not representative of Egyptian women since only those with at least one child aged 6–71 months were included in the study. A criterion for anaemia in non-pregnant women, whether lactating or not, is a haemoglobin value below 12 g. In pregnant women, it is a value less than 11 g (WHO, 1968). Anaemia was highest among lactating mothers (25.3 per cent), followed by pregnant mothers (22.1 per cent) and non-pregnant mothers (17.0 per cent). Overall prevalence among women was 22.4 per cent.

Other scattered surveys focusing on health centres, rather than community, reveal a much higher prevalence of iron deficiency anaemia.

## Other Micronutrient Deficiencies in Egypt

Some deficiencies observed in Egypt are not considered public health problems. Rickets and deficiencies of vitamin A, riboflavin, and zinc fall within this group.

Iodine deficiency disorders (IDD), manifested by goitre, caused serious affliction in the New Valley (Abdou, 1965), where iodization of salt showed remarkable results. In other parts of Egypt, the prevalence of IDD did not exceed 10 per cent. Recent data from a community-based survey on school children aged 6–18 years, in 24 governorates, revealed that IDD manifesting itself in the form of goitre, mostly grades IA & B, are prevalent among 38 per cent in the New Valley, 14 per cent in Souhag in Upper Egypt, and less than 10 per cent in all other governorates (Aly *et al.*, 1981).

## OBESITY

The association between obesity and diabetes, hypertension, cardiovascular disease, some types of cancer, and reduced life expectancy is a generally accepted reality (WHO, 1989, 1990). For these reasons, the prevalence of obesity in the general population is a rough indication of the health status of the population.

Obesity, resulting from energy overconsumption beyond actual physiological needs, is an emerging problem in Egypt. Obesity is diagnosed when weight-for-height is 120 per cent or more of the reference standard, or the body mass index (BMI) is 30 or more in adults. However, weight monitoring should detect the stage of overweight when weight-for-height is 110–<120 per cent of the reference standard, and BMI is 25–<30 where prevention of obesity is much easier than treatment of an already established case.

Table 8.3 shows prevalence of overweight and obesity in different age groups in Egypt. Among pre-schoolers the highest rate was registered in Cairo (18.3 per cent) followed by urban areas (14.8 per cent) and rural areas (13.9 per cent). In a five-year period, obesity has almost doubled, drawing attention to the need for proper nutrition orientation of mothers.

Among females in the age group 12 years till adulthood, the prevalence of overweight and obesity is rising, reaching its peak among mothers—63.1 per cent (Aly *et al.*, 1981). Earlier studies on school children in Cairo comparing data for 1962 (Abdou and Mahfouz, 1967a;

**Table 8.3** Prevalence of overweight and obesity[*] in different age groups in Egypt (National Studies, 1981 and 1984)

| Age group (years) | Males | Females | Total |
|---|---|---|---|
| <6 | — | — | 14.2 |
| 6–<12 | — | — | 10.9 |
| 12–<15 | 3.6 | 16.1 | 9.8 |
| 15–<18 | — | 21.6 | 10.8 |
| 18 + (unmarried) | 19.4 | 36.1 | 27.7 |
| Fathers and mothers | 14.5 | 63.1 | 38.8 |

[*] Weight-for-height 110% and more of WHO/NCHS Reference Standard for all age groups except <6 years where weight-for-age≥ 110% is used
Source: *National Food Consumption Study of Egypt* (Aly *et al.*, 1981) and HPE–HES (Moussa, 1988)

1968a) with that for 1975 (Aly *et al.*, 1980) revealed almost similar results as those of NFCS.

Both Sarhan (1982) and Habib (1987) carried out in-depth study on obese teenage schoolers (12–16 years) in Cairo and Ismailia, respectively. Rather similar results were obtained.

In general, the prevalence of obesity in Egypt is comparable with that in affluent countries of the Middle East, such as Saudi Arabia, Kuwait, and Iran. However, these rates are much higher than those in USA, which itself has more cases of obesity than northern European countries. The prevalence of adult obesity in USA in 1987, as defined by BMI, more than 25 was 26.7 per cent for women and 24.4 per cent for men in the age group 20–74 years (WHO, 1989). Unlike Egypt where obesity seems to be increasing, the prevalence rate in USA is almost unchanged from the rate determined by a survey conducted six years earlier.

It may be concluded that obesity is an emerging problem of public health importance in Egypt, requiring an urgent national programme for its prevention and control.

## FUNCTIONAL CONSEQUENCES OF MALNUTRITION

The functional consequences of the two main nutritional problems in Egypt, namely, PEM and iron deficiency anaemia, can be summarized by their effects on physical growth, immunocompetence and morbidity, cognitive function and social behaviour, work performance, reproduction, and lactation. This complex topic has been studied in Egypt in two main research projects: the Collaborative Research Support Program (CRSP) on food intake and human functions (Galal *et al.*, 1987; Calloway *et al.*, 1988) as well as anaemia and human functions (Hussein *et al.*, 1988). Positive correlation was found between energy, protein intake, as well as iron status and human functions. In all the three CRSP projects, conducted in Egypt, Kenya, and Mexico (Calloway *et al.*, 1988), body size characteristics of infants and toddlers correlated with measures of mental development. Bigger children scored better and were more socially active while smaller children were more prone to illness.

## DIET RELATED CHRONIC NON-COMMUNICABLE DISEASES

The main examples of these diet-related diseases are diabetes mellitus, cardiovascular disease, and cancer.

## Diabetes Mellitus (DM)

Diabetes mellitus (DM) is of two types: type I and type II. Although both types are treated wholly, or at least in part, by dietary measures, the cause of type II diabetes appears to be more directly related to dietary factors, namely, obesity. Often it is called non-insulin dependent diabetes, although insulin is occasionally used as a last resort. About 80 per cent of all type II diabetics are obese (WHO, 1989). Obesity is believed to contribute to the insulin resistance of this type of diabetes, and the best prevention known for diabetes would be the reduction of obesity in a given population.

During the HPE–HIS (Said, 1987), the awareness rate for self-reported diabetes was 13.2/1000 persons interviewed. Of diabetics aware of their deficiency, 19.4 per cent were current smokers—a rate that was applicable for urban as well as rural areas. However, there were more smokers among male diabetics (43.2 per cent) than among female diabetics (4.0 per cent)..More than half the diabetic smokers (50–60 per cent) smoked 10–20 cigarettes per day, regardless of area and sex.

Studies on diabetes control in different socio-economic groups (Rihan and Lebshtein, 1971) revealed that success in the control of diabetes depends more on the patient's cooperation in following the prescribed diet, rather than supplying him with drugs. This emphasizes the value, and the need for, a special nutrition and health education programme for diabetics of low socio-economic backgrounds.

## Cardiovascular Disease

Extensive and convincing evidence has been accumulated linking diet to serum lipid concentration and to atherosclerosis. Many dietary factors, such as the amount and kind of fat, the content and type of carbohydrate and protein, the presence of vitamins, minerals, and fibre have been reported to influence serum lipid concentration. Hypertension and coronary heart disease occur as a sequel to atherogenesis.

During the HPE–HIS, the awareness rate for self-reported hypertension and heart disease were 15.8 and 10.7 per 1000 persons interviewed, respectively. The male–female ratios were 0.4 and 0.7, respectively. Among those who suffered from hypertension, or had heart ailments, 17 per cent and 18 per cent respectively were current cigarette smokers, a greater number being male than female. About 70 per cent of these addicts smoked 10–20 cigarettes per day.

During HPE–HES, blood pressure was measured for a sample of 14,151 persons above the age of 6 years, including 48.0 per cent female and 33.7 per cent from urban areas. Systolic hypertension above 150 mm Hg was found among 113.4 per 1000 persons, while diastolic hypertension was prevalent among 47.4 per 1000. Hypertension prevalence, mainly a problem of adulthood and old age, was found to increase by age. Systolic hypertension was more frequent among urban residents. Urbanization and its subsequent stress syndrome, and changes in environment, food intake, and habits such as smoking are major risk factors. As will be discussed later in this chapter, there has been an increase in the consumption of energy, animal fat, and sugar in the period 1965–85.

## Cancer

Descriptive statistics of the National Cancer Institute, Cairo, were presented by many investigators at the Symposium on Nutrition and Cancer, organized by the Egyptian Nutrition Society in 1981. These confirm the high frequency of bladder cancer, followed by breast cancer, the commonest neoplasm in females. Malignancy of lymphatic and haemopoietic system ranks next, together with malignancy of the digestive organs. Statistics show low frequency of colon cancer and relatively high frequency of rectal cancer. The lowest incidence is cancer of the buccal cavity and pharynx. Figure 8.2 shows the distribution of cases registered (according to sex) by the Cancer Registry for the Metropolitan Cairo Area (Sherif and Ibrahim, 1988).

Breast cancer could be related to starchy diet and overweight, in other words, total energy intake. Nitrosamine production could be traced to a high nitrite content in diet, possibly due to contamination from fertilizers. This is related to the aetiology of bladder cancer, and possibly hypopharyngeal cancer.

Vitamin A deficiency might play a role in the relatively high frequency of squamous cell carcinoma. Bilharzial patients showed a significantly low level of vitamin A, retinol, and beta-carotenes as compared with normal subjects. The Egyptian diet can hinder certain digestive tract cancers, possibly due to its high fibre and rich vitamin C content.

Animal studies showed that restricting energy intake generally inhibits development of most kinds of tumours, particularly mammary tumours. They showed also that increasing the level of fat in diet stimulates mammary tumour development (WHO, 1989). This suggests that dietary fat acts as a promoting agent, producing a more favourable

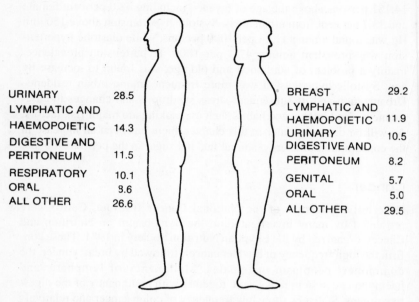

| URINARY | 28.5 |
| LYMPHATIC AND HAEMOPOIETIC | 14.3 |
| DIGESTIVE AND PERITONEUM | 11.5 |
| RESPIRATORY | 10.1 |
| ORAL | 9.6 |
| ALL OTHER | 26.6 |

| BREAST | 29.2 |
| LYMPHATIC AND HAEMOPOIETIC | 11.9 |
| URINARY | 10.5 |
| DIGESTIVE AND PERITONEUM | 8.2 |
| GENITAL | 5.7 |
| ORAL | 5.0 |
| ALL OTHER | 29.5 |

**Fig. 8.2.** Site distribution of cases registered by the cancer registry for the Metropolitan Cairo area, according to sex

environment for the development of latent tumour cells. Unsaturated fats seem to be inductive than saturated fats in promoting mammary tumorigenesis.

Dietary factors are considered as modifiers, rather than initiators, of tumorigenesis. Heavy metals, which may enter the body via food and drinking water, are potential dietary carcinogens. Dietary trace element imbalance is sometimes associated with a high risk of certain types of cancer. Both deficiency and excess of a particular trace element can be carcinogenic.

## MAJOR DETERMINANTS OF NUTRITIONAL STATUS OF THE POPULATION 'ENVIRONMENT'

As the causes of malnutrition are multidimensional, policies formulated for countering malnutrition should also be multidimensional. Apart from the targeted, short-term, appropriate nutrition intervention programmes, accelerated agricultural and economic development will provide the only long-term solution.

In order to be effective, agricultural development, as well as targeted nutrition intervention programmes, should be based on proper information on per caput food supplies and per caput food consumption as well as macro-economic environment and health status. Changes in per caput food supplies result from changes in food production, net food import, feed and seed uses, food stocks, and changes in population. The relation between food prices and earnings is largely influenced by food supply.

## MACRO-ECONOMIC ENVIRONMENT AND NUTRITION

### Urban and Rural Consumer Prices

Index numbers of urban and rural prices are one of the most important indicators of the inflation in food prices and its subsequent negative impacts on the poor. According to official data (CAPMAS, 1991), the food and beverages index of urban consumer prices increased from 100.0 in 1966–67 to 1839.8 in 1990. The index of rural consumer prices also increased from 100.0 to 1822.5 in the same period. This steep rise in food prices had a significant impact on real income, particularly that of the poor. In Egypt it was found that 10 per cent increase in food prices led to 5.6 per cent decrease in the real income of the low-income groups, the lowest 10 per cent (Pinstrup-Andersen, 1987).

Prices of many basic food products sharply increased in 1990 from January to December. The majority of the high increases covers the rationed and public sector products: rationed rice has increased by 75 per cent, and rationed vegetable oil by 89 per cent.

### Behaviour of Families vis-a-vis Rising Food Prices

Retail prices for all food commodities have increased dramatically during the period 1975 to 1985–86. The family budget survey of 1981–82, conducted by CAPMAS, showed that 51 per cent and 53.3 per cent of per capita expenditure in urban and rural areas respectively are spent on food. An estimate of the lowest expenses on balanced diet for the average Egyptian family was conducted by Egypt's NI, using the price list of food commodities in 1981, 1984, and 1989 (Hussein, 1989). The cost of the minimum food basket registered an increase of 429 per cent for urban and 391 per cent for rural Egyptian families from 1981–82 to 1989. This rise in the cost of food is considered too high in comparison with the comparatively lower rise in salaries.

A study was conducted by the NI on a sample of 350 households (HHs) representing Cairo, a governorate from upper and another from lower Egypt, as well as an industrial area (Hussein, 1989). Results revealed the following data:

— rise in income does not cope with rise in food cost;
— consumption of less expensive foods as a substitute for more expensive ones, without consideration of the loss in nutritive value, compromised both quantity and quality of the diet;
— the higher the level of education within the HH, the higher was the sum of expenditure on food;
— low frequency of meat consumption was generally favoured.

## Structural Adjustment

Egypt entered a critical period when it was faced with difficulties in covering its debt service obligations and a negative net resource transfer. In the summer of 1986, the government prepared a macro-economic reform programme, which served as a base for the 1987/88–1991/92 second development plan and the stand-by agreement with the International Monetary Fund (IMF) in May 1987. Since 1987 a number of reform measures in the economic policy at the macro-level were implemented, bringing about major changes in prices and subsidies. Then, the Egyptian government began to strengthen and accelerate its reform measures in 1989, with direct repercussions on its exchange rate policies, privatization, pricing policies, and social policies.

Various reform measures include energy prices and electricity tariffs, which were increased to international standards. Water charges, telephone and railway tariffs, car insurance fees, and prices of many industrial goods were raised to cover production costs. The most striking feature of this reform era is the decrease in the consumer goods subsidies and the establishment of a free exchange market. Customs tariffs were modified, quantitative import restrictions were reduced, and exports were, to a large extent, encouraged and liberalized. The combined effect of these efforts on the lives of the underprivileged remains to be seen.

# FOOD SECURITY

A scrutiny of both production and consumption of some food crops by the Ministry of Agriculture in 1991 disclosed that certain crops such as maize, rice, potatoes, onions, citrus fruits, melons, and water melons are in surplus, whereas wheat production does not meet the demand for consumption. The reason for this escalation in consumption beyond the production levels may be traced primarily to the soaring growth in population. Also, the rise in income levels reflected the type and amount of consumption during the last decade.

## Trends of Food Supply in Egypt in the Last 20 Years

The Food Balance Sheets (FBS) of 1965 and 1985 were compared for certain food items and selected nutrients related mostly to the emerging category of diet-related, chronic, non-communicable diseases. Comparative studies revealed that availability of meat and milk increased by almost 50 per cent whereas that of sugar more than doubled, and that of animal fat almost doubled. Total energy consumption has increased by almost 50 per cent (Table 8.4).

The obvious increase in all animal foods, sugar, as well as total energy, animal protein, and animal fat is not desirable from the health point of view, indicating the need for targeted action towards prevention of diet-related, chronic, non-communicable diseases.

## Contribution of Selected Food Groups to Dietary Energy Supply (DES)

Cereals—mainly wheat, rice and, to a lesser extent, corn—are the main contributors to DES in Egypt. This is evident from the series of FBSs from 1969 to 1986 (Ministry of Agriculture, 1991) when cereals supplied from 61.6 per cent to 79.5 per cent of DES. They are also the main contributors to protein supply.

Legumes, mainly lentils and fava beans, which are popular substitutes for animal protein sources in Egypt, did not supply more than 5.4 per cent of DES (1969) and only 3.6 per cent in 1986. The percentage contribution of the total animal products to DES ranged from 8.9 per cent to 11.4 per cent with minor fluctuations and a perceptible drop since 1984.

NFCS and other studies showed variation of nutrient intake with the following factors: Energy intake is slightly higher in rural than urban

**Table 8.4** Trends of food availability in Egypt within a 18-year period. Food Balance Sheets (FBS) 1969-86

| Per caput/day | 1969 | 1970 | 1971 | 1972 | 1973 | 1974 | 1975 | 1976 | 1977 | 1978 | 1979 | 1980 | 1981 | 1982 | 1983 | 1984 | 1985 | 1986 |
|---|---|---|---|---|---|---|---|---|---|---|---|---|---|---|---|---|---|---|
| Total calories (Kcal) | 2660 | 2891 | 2747 | 2744 | 2833 | 3142 | 3394 | 3340 | 3360 | 3052 | 3343 | 3386 | 3774 | 3562 | 3521 | 3599 | 3745 | 3501 |
| Dietary energy supply (DES) | | | | | | | | | | | | | | | | | | |
| Total protein (g) | 74.6 | 82 | 76.9 | 75.7 | 78.8 | 87.2 | 93.4 | 91.9 | 91.7 | 94.9 | 91.5 | 95.5 | 106.7 | 98.2 | 98.4 | 102.3 | 103 | 90.6 |
| Animal | 10.6 | 10.7 | 10.6 | 10.6 | 10.5 | 10.8 | 11 | 12.5 | 11.9 | 13.3 | 11.5 | 14.5 | 15.5 | 14 | 15.1 | 13.6 | 13.9 | 14 |
| Plant | 64 | 71.3 | 66.3 | 65.1 | 68.3 | 76.4 | 82.4 | 79.4 | 79.8 | 81.6 | 80 | 81 | 91.2 | 84.2 | 83.3 | 88.7 | 89.1 | 76.6 |
| Total fat (g) | 48.8 | 47.1 | 46.1 | 48 | 47.1 | 53.2 | 61.3 | 61 | 61.5 | 65.4 | 59.8 | 56 | 64.3 | 62.5 | 62.2 | 54.4 | 70.3 | 78.2 |
| Animal | 12.3 | 11 | 11.9 | 11.7 | 11.7 | 11.8 | 12.3 | 14.1 | 13.9 | 14.1 | 13.8 | 15.5 | 16 | 15.1 | 15.7 | 14.5 | 13.7 | 13.7 |
| Plant | 36.5 | 36.1 | 34.2 | 36.3 | 35.4 | 41.4 | 49 | 46.9 | 47.6 | 51.3 | 46 | 40.5 | 48.3 | 47.4 | 46.5 | 39.9 | 56.6 | 64.5 |

Source: Serial food Balance Sheets of Egypt (Ministry of Agriculture, 1991)

areas. However, animal protein is much higher in urban areas (29.2 g) than in rural areas (19.6 g). The difference in energy intake between seasons is minimal; but it is slightly lower in summer, the hottest season of the year.

In spite of the increased requirements of energy, and macro- and micronutrients of both pregnant and lactating mothers, the usual behaviour of mothers registers no change in quantity or quality of diet with resulting to dietary inadequacy (Galal *et al.*, 1987; Abdel Ghany, 1986; Girgis, 1987). In the case of smaller families, the per caput intake of both energy and animal protein was found to be higher than the per caput intake in larger families (Aly *et al.*, 1981). From the demographic data obtained through WHO/EMRO (1991), the national figure for the average family size was 5.0 in 1976 and 4.9 in 1986. This finding emphasizes the need for extra efforts in the area of family planning.

## Adequacy of Egyptian Diets

From the NFCS (Aly *et al.*, 1981) it was observed that energy is more inadequate than protein, both in adults and dependent family members in the age group 2–18 years; energy and protein deficiency are more prevalent in urban than rural areas and more common among fathers than mothers.

More recent data derived from a longitudinal study of a rural community revealed the same trend with respect to energy and protein adequacy. However, inadequacy of micronutrients was more prominent than that of energy and protein.

In fact, energy and protein are supplied mainly by bread, the lowcost, main staple in Egypt. Iron inadequacy was maximum among mothers, almost two-thirds of whose iron consumption does not satisfy 90 per cent of the specified RDA (WHO, 1974, 1989). Almost one-third of pre-schoolers get less than 90 per cent of their iron RDA. Less than 5 per cent of fathers and almost 10 per cent of schoolers (7–9 years) have diets inadequate in iron.

The diet of family members was inadequate in vitamin A although manifest clinical signs were lacking. An in-depth study for vitamin A status in Egypt is needed for a complete record of dietary patterns.

## INFANT AND CHILD FEEDING

Research on feeding practices of children under two years of age have revealed important differences between rural and urban populations and between the general urban population and the less privileged population of Cairo, Giza, and Alexandria. Children in rural areas are exclusively breast-fed longer and completely weaned at a later age than the general population of urban children. The pattern of feeding in early childhood in the less privileged, urban families is closer to the rural pattern than the general urban practices. These differences suggest that, among rural and less privileged urban mothers, traditional patterns remain influential, or the availability of weaning foods, either actual or in terms of cost, is less.

Three other studies arrive at rather similar conclusions. More than two-thirds of infants at one year of age are still breast-fed, and 30 per cent approaching their second year continue to be breast-fed. Breast-feeding for more than two years is uncommon: less than 10 per cent (ARE–NSS, 1978; Moussa et al., 1988a; Sayed et al., 1989).

## Weaning Foods

During the weaning period, the young child diet changes from milk alone to the regular family diet. The prevailing types of weaning foods, consumed by almost two-thirds of Egyptian children, belong predominantly to five categories—mammalian milk and milk products, portion of family diet, preparations such as biscuits, and other processed cereals. However, only about one-fifth of the children consume, during the weaning period, a diet specially prepared daily for the child or commercially-prepared weaning foods. During the first six months of the infant's life, home-prepared cereals, mostly wheat and rice, as well as starch puddings are favoured.

In some rural areas of Egypt, infants are fed water and sugar. New weaning foods are gradually introduced, and by the age of 18–24 months more varieties are used by a higher percentage of children. These include legumes, tubers, fats and oils, eggs, meat or chicken, vegetables, and fruits. The ability of the child's diet (less than 2 years of age) to satisfy his RDA of energy and protein, based on recommended dietary allowances of FAO/WHO/UNU (1985), was compared with percentage RDA per caput in the same child's family. The study revealed that 53.8 per cent of children and 31.8 per cent of their families do not satisfy the RDA for energy and protein, respectively, while for almost one-third of cases the family diet satisfies per caput energy RDA but not the child. For this group, nutrition education should prove beneficial, as food is available in the home, but the mother is unaware of the child's needs.

Those parents who give more care to the child than to themselves are in a minority not exceeding 14 per cent (Moussa *et al.*, 1988; Moussa, 1990).

One of the main factors causing inadequate diet for infants during the weaning period is that the food composition is mostly part of the family diet which is predominantly vegetarian, with a high amount of dietary fibre. The study revealed that the majority of children less than two years of age get diets with less energy density and less protein energy ratio than that of their families (Moussa *et al.*, 1988b; Moussa, 1990).

The available energy and protein utilization of normal home diets was investigated in a nitrogen balance study, covering six completely weaned pre-school children in a rural Egyptian community (Moussa *et al.*, 1989). The results were compared with an earlier study of children who were fed three well-balanced diets (Moussa, 1973; Abdou *et al.*, 1975). Figure 8.3 shows apparent digestibility and net protein utilization (NPU) of the four types of diets. A typical rural diet of toddlers was seen to have values much lower than the other three balanced diets. Supramine and Sesamena which are mainly mixtures of cereals and legumes, with 10 per cent dried skimmed milk (DSM) in the former and 10 per cent dehulled sesame (tehineh) in the latter, have values quite comparable to the milk formula. These results have important implica-

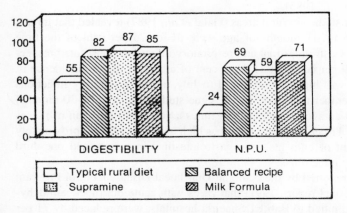

**Fig. 8.3** Energy and protein bioavailability of different diets fed to children during 72-hour metabolic periods
Source: Weaning Foods (Moussa, 1990)

tions in the nutrition education messages to mothers, whether through the Primary Health Care (PHC) system or through social marketing techniques.

## SANITATION, HEALTH BEHAVIOUR, AND INFECTION

The percentage of population covered by safe water supply in Egypt in 1982 was 100 in urban and 49 in rural areas. The proportion in the rural areas has improved to 90 per cent in 1987. The percentage of the population covered by adequate sanitary facilities (sewage disposal mainly) was 95 in urban areas and 42 in rural areas in 1982, and improved to 100 and 65 respectively during 1987 (WHO/EMRO, 1991). This should reduce infection.

The morbidity load in Egypt, particularly in pre-school children, is indicated mainly by diarrhoea and respiratory infections, as proved by statistics from the Ministry of Health as well as many community-based research studies. Detailed studies on urban children under the age of 3 years revealed that diarrhoea was the cause of morbidity in 37.7 per cent of cases in under-privileged areas in Cairo, and 24.7 per cent in Alexandria, whereas respiratory infections were responsible for 29.4 per cent and 36.4 per cent of cases respectively. The nutritional status was better in areas where the incidence of diarrhoea was lower. In Cairo, children suffered 13 per cent of the time from diarrhoea in a three-month period (Moussa *et al.*, 1983).

Similar studies in rural areas (Galal *et al.*, 1987) revealed that infants from birth to six months of age were ill for 25 per cent of the time observed. Gastrointestinal and respiratory infections constituted respectively 37.9 per cent and 31.8 per cent of all infant illness. Incidence of diarrhoea was highest from April to July, and of respiratory infections from December to March. In the same study, toddlers (18–30 months) fell ill, on an average, almost ten times a year, the time span of illness averaging 11 per cent but ranging as high as 30 per cent. Approximately 40 per cent of ailments were gastrointestinal in nature, and one-third respiratory infections.

It was reported by the National Diarrhoeal Disease Control Program (NDDCP, final report, 1991) that cases with acute diarrhoea and dehydration, admitted to Bab El Shaeiria hospitals, were reduced by 71 per cent in 1984 and up to 75 per cent in 1990. Also, the percentage of mothers who stopped breast-feeding during diarrhoea was reduced from

58 per cent in 1980 to 5 per cent in 1988. A considerable impact on the nutritional status of pre-school age children is thus expected.

## Parasitic Infestation

The relation of parasites and malnutrition was studied in the HPE–HES (Moussa, 1988a) covering school children aged 6–12 years, in different nutritional grades, based on weight-for-age categories. The investigation revealed the following data (Table 8.5):

**Table 8.5** Prevalence of parasities among Schoolers (6–12 years) of Different Classes of Nutritional Status, Whole Sample

| Nutritional status Wt/Age % of median | Sex | Positive for parasites | | | | | |
|---|---|---|---|---|---|---|---|
| | | Urine Bilh. | Intes Bilh. | Ancylo-stoma | Asca-ris | Amo-eba | Total |
| 3rd degree | M | 21.6 | 0.0 | 7.8 | 3.9 | 5.9 | 51 |
| undernutrition | F | 22.7 | 0.0 | 4.0 | 9.3 | 5.3 | 75 |
| <60 | T | 22.2 | 0.0 | 5.6 | 7.1 | 5.6 | 126 |
| 2nd degree | M | 16.6 | 0.6 | 2.2 | 6.8 | 4.4 | 362 |
| undernutrition | F | 7.9 | 0.6 | 2.5 | 13.0 | 6.2 | 354 |
| 60–74.9 | T | 12.3 | 0.6 | 2.4 | 10.9 | 5.3 | 716 |
| 1st degree | M | 16.4 | 0.0 | 1.7 | 11.5 | 4.5 | 706 |
| undernutrition | F | 8.7 | 0.0 | 3.4 | 20.2 | 6.0 | 587 |
| 75–89.9 | T | 12.9 | 0.0 | 2.5 | 10.8 | 5.2 | 1293 |
| Normal | M | 11.6 | 0.0 | 1.5 | 9.9 | 3.1 | 413 |
| weight | F | 8.4 | 0.0 | 1.7 | 9.4 | 4.2 | 406 |
| 90–109.9 | T | 10.0 | 0.0 | 1.6 | 9.6 | 3.7 | 819 |
| overweight | M | 18.4 | 0.0 | 0.0 | 8.2 | 4.1 | 49 |
| 110–119.9 | F | 12.9 | 0.0 | 0.0 | 11.3 | 8.1 | 62 |
| | T | 15.3 | 0.0 | 0.0 | 9.9 | 6.3 | 111 |
| Obese | M | 17.5 | 3.2 | 1.6 | 14.3 | 1.6 | 63 |
| | F | 5.6 | 4.2 | 0.0 | 8.5 | 5.6 | 71 |
| 120+ | T | 11.2 | 3.7 | 0.7 | 11.2 | 3.7 | 134 |
| | M | 15.5 | 0.4 | 1.9 | 10.3 | 4.1 | 1647 |
| Total | F | 9.1 | 0.4 | 2.5 | 10.5 | 5.6 | 1556 |
| | T | 12.4 | 0.4 | 2.2 | 10.4 | 4.8 | 3203 |
| Cairo | M | 0.0 | 0.0 | 0.0 | 1.4 | 3.5 | 141 |
| sample | F | 0.0 | 0.0 | 0.0 | 3.7 | 8.8 | 136 |
| | T | 0.0 | 0.0 | 0.0 | 2.5 | 6.1 | 277 |

Source: *Nutritional Status in Egypt, Health Profile of Egypt* (Moussa, 1988a)

— Urinary bilharziasis was most prevalent among the group of third-degree undernutrition and least prevalent among the group of normal weight-for-age. This may be attributed to the effect of ecology and quality of life on both the prevalence of parasites and nutritional status. There were more victims of urinary bilharziasis in almost all groups, which is mostly due to more exposure. The overall prevalence of urinary bilharziasis in the whole sample of Egypt ($n$=3203) was 12.4 per cent. In the small sample of Cairo ($n$=277), it was zero; only 0.4 per cent of school-age children were infected with intestinal bilharziasis.

— Ancylostoma is also more prevalent in the group of third-degree undernutrition (<60 per cent wt/age of reference median), the overall prevalence being 2.2 per cent.

— The incidence of ascariasis was highest among the overweight group (but not exceeding 15 per cent). The fact that the highest level was observed among obese, school-age children points to the greater likelihood of infection with greater consumption of food.

— Amoebiasis was least prevalent among the group of normal weight-for-age while the highest incidence was among the overweight group.

The prevalence of parasites was also studied among anaemic subjects by age and sex. For the sample for Egypt (6 years and above), see Table 8.6. Prevalence of parasitic infestations among the whole sample group—anaemic and non-anaemic—was less for all types of parasites. The incidence of parasitic infestation in the Cairo sample was much less than in the whole sample. The general trend is a decrease in the parasitic load in the last decade, particularly ancylostomiasis and bilharziasis.

## CARING CAPACITY WITHIN THE HOUSEHOLD

Studies of Egyptian households showed that the knowledge, attitudes, and practices of family members, particularly of the household head and the primary care provider, largely determine the nutritional status of the household. In many cases, malnutrition is attributable to lack of understanding of the body's food needs. This was proven by results concerned with infant feeding and weaning practices wherein almost one-third of the sample, food was available in the household but the child did not get his RDA of energy and protein (Moussa *et al.*, 1988b; Moussa, 1990).

Research has found maternal education level, independent of house-

**Table 8.6** Prevalence of parasites among Anaemic Subjects by Age and Sex, Whole Sample (6+ years)

| Age in years | Hb level | Sex | Positive for parasites | | | | | |
|---|---|---|---|---|---|---|---|---|
| | | | Urine Bilh. | Intes Bilh. | Ancylo-stoma | Asca-ris | Amo-eba | Total |
| 6– | <12 | M | 11.9 | 0.0 | 2.5 | 10.4 | 4.0 | 530 |
| | <12 | F | 8.7 | 0.0 | 2.8 | 10.4 | 5.5 | 530 |
| | | T | 10.3 | 0.0 | 2.6 | 10.4 | 4.7 | 1060 |
| 10– | <12 | M | 25.2 | 0.3 | 3.5 | 9.8 | 4.0 | 579 |
| | <12 | F | 12.5 | 0.4 | 3.8 | 10.5 | 6.0 | 503 |
| | | T | 19.3 | 0.4 | 3.6 | 10.2 | 4.9 | 1082 |
| 15– | <13 | M | 25.1 | 0.0 | 3.9 | 6.5 | 5.5 | 490 |
| | <12 | F | 9.7 | 0.0 | 3.1 | 7.1 | 5.2 | 382 |
| | | T | 18.3 | 0.0 | 3.6 | 6.8 | 5.4 | 872 |
| 20– | <13 | M | 11.2 | 1.2 | 10.6 | 4.4 | 6.2 | 160 |
| | <12 | F | 4.7 | 0.0 | 2.1 | 7.1 | 4.0 | 524 |
| | | T | 8.3 | 0.3 | 4.1 | 6.4 | 4.5 | 684 |
| 30– | <13 | M | 9.6 | 0.0 | 2.4 | 6.4 | 4.8 | 125 |
| | <12 | F | 3.6 | 0.0 | 2.7 | 8.9 | 6.0 | 414 |
| | | T | 5.0 | 0.0 | 2.6 | 8.3 | 5.8 | 539 |
| 40– | <13 | M | 8.6 | 1.7 | 3.4 | 7.8 | 6.0 | 116 |
| | <12 | F | 2.8 | 0.0 | 1.4 | 6.6 | 6.2 | 289 |
| | | T | 4.4 | 0.5 | 2.0 | 6.9 | 6.2 | 405 |
| 50– | <13 | M | 5.8 | 0.0 | 6.5 | 4.3 | 7.2 | 138 |
| | <12 | F | 3.1 | 0.0 | 1.0 | 7.9 | 4.7 | 191 |
| | | T | 4.3 | 0.0 | 3.3 | 6.4 | 5.8 | 329 |
| 60– | <13 | M | 1.1 | 0.0 | 2.2 | 4.9 | 4.4 | 182 |
| | <12 | F | 0.0 | 0.0 | 0.0 | 0.0 | 0.0 | 0 |
| | | T | 1.1 | 0.0 | 2.2 | 4.9 | 4.4 | 182 |
| | | M | 16.5 | 0.3 | 3.8 | 7.9 | 4.8 | 2320 |
| Total | | F | 7.6 | 0.1 | 2.6 | 8.6 | 5.4 | 2833 |
| | | T | 11.6 | 0.2 | 3.2 | 8.3 | 5.1 | 5153 |
| Cairo | | M | 0.0 | 0.0 | 0.0 | 1.6 | 4.7 | 64 |
| sample | | F | 0.0 | 0.0 | 0.0 | 1.6 | 5.6 | 126 |
| | | T | 0.0 | 0.0 | 0.0 | 1.6 | 5.3 | 190 |

Source: *Nutritional Status in Egypt, Health Profile of Egypt* (Moussa, 1988a)

hold income, to be positively related to better nutritional status of children and to lower infant mortality. Maternal time-allocation studies revealed that education of mothers was positively associated with the time they devoted to child care (Noor *et al.*, 1991). In the low-income sample of mostly uneducated mothers (Moussa *et al.*, 1988b), only around one-tenth of mothers gave more care to the child than the rest of the household members. In Egypt, the adult literacy rate (10 years and above) was 56 per cent for males and 28 per cent for females in 1980. It increased to 62 per cent and 38 per cent respectively in 1987. The urban–rural ratio of 60:29 increased to only 61:35 in 1987 (WHO/EMRO, 1991).

In the DHS (Sayed *et al.*, 1988), it was found that one-third of the sample children who had suffered from diarrhoea for seven days were not given any treatment. Mothers did not seek medical advice in spite of available health services, the proportion of such negligence being highest in rural areas, especially in Upper Egypt (40.5 per cent) and lowest among mothers working for cash (18.1 per cent). These results call for intensive education in general health and nutrition.

## Accessibility and Utilization of Health Services

Accessibility and utilization of health services is a critical determinant of the health and nutritional status of populations. In Egypt, there is an excellent primary health care (PHC) network of facilities, adequately staffed with qualified personnel. The services have improved from 1981 to 1988, and in 1990 the coverage by physicians and nurses was even higher. The MOH opened new nursing schools in the last few years in order to overcome the nursing shortage. However, the ratio between physicians and nurses in the health team needs further correction.

The DHS (Sayed *et al.*, 1988) shows that the percentage of fully immunized children (12–23 months) is highest in the urban governorates, which utilize the free available services better than Upper Egyptians who make the least use of the health services. In spite of free available health services to cover maternal care, about one-half of pregnant women have a pre-natal check-up, about one-fifth have their babies delivered in hospitals or clinics, and one-tenth have tetanus injections.

Infant and child mortality rates are sensitive indicators of the impact of health and nutrition services. Table 8.7 shows the trends of neonatal, post neonatal, infant mortality rate (IMR) and child (1–4 years) mortality rates during the period 1976–88 (CAPMAS, 1991). There is marked improvement in post-neonatal mortality rates. The distinct drop in IMR since 1984 is attributed to NDDCP and the Expanded Programme of Immunization (EPI).

**Table 8.7** Neo-natal, Post-neonatal and Infant Mortality during 1976–88

| Years | Neo-natal | Post-neonatal | IMR | CMR |
|-------|-----------|---------------|------|------|
| 1976 | 14.9 | 72.6 | 87.5 | 17.3 |
| 1977 | 14.8 | 70.5 | 85.3 | 18.0 |
| 1978 | 13.8 | 59.7 | 73.3 | 12.5 |
| 1979 | 12.2 | 64.2 | 76.4 | 16.5 |
| 1980 | 14.4 | 61.6 | 76.0 | 10.8 |
| 1981 | 12.2 | 58.1 | 70.3 | 10.9 |
| 1982 | 14.9 | 55.6 | 70.5 | 13.0 |
| 1983 | 12.4 | 52.2 | 64.6 | 9.3 |
| 1984 | 12.3 | 49.8 | 62.1 | 10.0 |
| 1985 | 11.6 | 37.7 | 49.3 | 9.3 |
| 1986 | 13.1 | 34.0 | 47.1 | 7.5 |
| 1987 | 13.4 | 36.0 | 49.4 | 7.5 |
| 1988 | 12.7 | 30.6 | 43.3 | 6.7 |

Source: CAPMAS, Statistical Department, Annual Report of Vital Statistics, 1976–88

## CURRENT POLICIES. PROGRAMMES, AND INTERVENTIONS FOR PROMOTION OF NUTRITIONAL STATUS

The MOH bears the main responsibility for interventions directed towards improving the health and nutritional status of the Egyptians. There are also a lot of interventions, policies, and programmes carried out by other institutions, ministries, and non-governmental organizations (NGOs) aiming at the same goal. The ministries of Agriculture, Economics, Planning, Industry, Social Affairs, Education, and Supplies implement programmes which are geared to the nutritional and health status of the population.

The main projects aiming to improve nutrition have been related to food subsidies, foreign aid, and nutrition education and communication. Other interventions that have contributed to nutrition are the family planning programme, school feeding programmes, enhanced agricultural production, EPI and the NDDCP.

### Food Subsidy Programme

Food rations, which were introduced during the Second World War, and continued up to the year 1965, were an outcome of the prevailing chronic food shortage. Food ration cards provided edible oil, sugar, tea, and kerosene.

During 1965, the Government of Egypt restructured its food ration cards, adding a few basic foods, such as wheat flour, and rice, and government cooperatives began to sell subsidized meat. eggs. chicken, and fish. At present this system has been terminated. A dramatic increase in the subsidy bill occurred after 1973, when world food prices rose steeply, multiplying several-fold the difference between actual costs and the low sale price of large amounts of food imports. Despite the downward trend in food prices in the late seventies, the food subsidy payments kept increasing, along with rising amounts of food imports and a falling exchange rate. The food subsidy cost in 1984–85 escalated to about L.E. 1.8 billion due to some major factors:

— rising per capita income, because of emigrant remittances;
— high rate of population growth;
— changing consumption patterns;
— relatively cheap price of subsidized balady bread.

During 1988–89 the ration/subsidy system has been modified in order to reduce costs to approximately half that of the 1984–85 programme. The cost-reduction measures have involved the following issues:

— raising ration/subsidy prices;
— reducing the number of items included in the system;
— reducing the quantities subsidized per person;
— increasing the balady bread price by 150 per cent during 1989;
— changing the mix of subsidized foods.

The increase in the price of bread and other basic commodities will penalize the low-income groups more than others, as food occupies a larger share of their total expenditure and bread provides 50–60 per cent of their energy. For these reasons, the Government of Egypt, on 1 May 1991, announced the establishment of the new 'Social Fund' with the purpose of limiting the impact of the economic reform policies on vulnerable sections of the population. This fund, with budgetary allocations earmarked at L.E. 1300 million by the end of 1992, will be financed mostly by foreign assistance.

## Foreign Aid (previously food aid)

For over 30 years, Egypt received aid in the form of food, medicine, clothing, and project finance, through international organizations, mainly the World Food Programme (WFP), and relief services such as CARE and Catholic Relief Services (CRS), as well as from donor countries such as Holland and Finland. The foods were mainly sources of energy and protein, usually enriched with vitamins and mineral salts. The main target groups were mothers and pre-school children; school children, particularly in rural areas; and new settlers on land reclamation projects (Aly *et al.*, 1976 and 1981).

The impact of wheat soya blend (WSB), donated by CRS to MCH centres for supplementary feeding, on the nutritional status of children under the age of 3 years was evaluated at the Rehabilitation Unit of the Nutrition Institute of Egypt, RUNI (Aly *et al.*, 1976). It was observed that the group fed WSB grew faster than the control group whose food was restricted to the traditional supplements.

Current assistance programmes are designed to eradicate dependence and promote self-reliance. This has been achieved by gradually substituting food aid through programmes which lead to socio-economic development; environmental sanitation and personal hygiene; improved health and nutritional awareness; and increased income. Such programmes enhance the capacity of the community to manage its own income-generating and health promotion programmes. To ensure sustainability in the long term, special attention is given to the technical and managerial capacity of a community or counterpart organization. At present, donors fund training programmes that will enable certain institutions to implement development projects.

## NUTRITION EDUCATION AND COMMUNICATION

### Mass Media

Dissemination of nutrition knowledge and health information via radio and television, newspapers, journals, and books has been an ongoing activity. Radio and T.V. sets are now installed in almost every urban and rural home. Of the mass media channels, T.V. is the most effective. Modern social marketing techniques have improved the quality of messages on topics ranging from the control of diarrhoea and diet during diarrhoeal attacks, to breast-feeding, immunization, family planning, and good nutrition and its importance to pregnant and nursing mothers. Information is disseminated through brief, effective spots and through in-depth programmes on health, women, and social programmes. The NI

staff members, as well as specialized university staff members, participate in all mass media campaigns. (See also Chapter 6.)

## Nutrition Education in Health Centres

In 1979, a project was designed to develop and test a nutrition education
programme that would strengthen the food and nutrition services extended via the Primary Health Care (PHC) network in Egypt. The project
planned to achieve that goal largely by educating mothers attending
MCH centres on nutrition, sanitation, health, and child care. The project
spanned three phases. During phase I, nutrition organizers from 18 governorates received a condensed training course on nutrition. They, in
turn, trained nurses working at PHC centres in these governorates. The
nutrition messages were directed mainly towards pre-school children
and the best use of food aid offered at these centres as well as the proper
use of growth charts and subsequent counselling.

In phase II of the project, nutrition education activities were expanded to cover most of the health centres in the same governorates. In
these two phases, the role of physicians was not specified, thereby causing a lack of support to nurses. This problem was eliminated in phase III,
where physicians were included in the training programme, and all the
nurses in each centre were trained as against one or two nurses in phases
I and II. The programme was designed to be implemented under the full
responsibility of the Health Directorate, with the NI as the technical
adviser.

In day-care centres, where nutrition education is now becoming an
integral component, teachers were trained in improving the nutritional
status of pre-schoolers. Teachers, in turn, transferred nutrition messages
to children, using untraditional methods, e.g. songs, plays, puppets.

## Nutrition Education in the School System and Health Programmes

In Egypt, nutrition education is integrated with many curricula for students (for example, science programmes include the nutrition component) as also in various health projects and programmes: NDDCP, the
Urban Health Development Programme, and the Strengthening Rural
Health Delivery Programme where nutrition education is a daily activity.

# POPULATION GROWTH, URBANIZATION, MIGRATION AND AGEING

## Population Growth

Egypt's population nearly doubled from 9.7 million to over 18 million persons in the 50 years from 1897 to 1947. The subsequent doubling took less than 30 years: from 1947 to 1976. The 1986 census of population, housing, and establishments placed the Egyptian population at 48.3 million. It is estimated that the total population multiplied to 57 million in 1991, and the expectation of life at birth has risen from 39 years in 1952 to over 60 years in the early 1990s (CAPMAS, 1991).

The population growth rate, which was 1.3 per cent annually at the beginning of this century, fell for a period. It began to rise rapidly from the early 1950s reaching a rate of approximately 2.7 per cent between the 1947 and 1960 censuses. For the period 1960–66, the growth rate decreased slightly to 2.5 per cent and continued dwindling to 1.9 per cent between 1966 and 1976. However, it increased again to nearly 2.8 per cent between the 1976 and 1986 censuses (CAPMAS, 1991).

## Urbanization and Migration

The geographic distribution of the Egyptian population clearly shows considerable human movement form rural to urban regions, resulting in high rates of urbanization and the concentration of the national population in prime cities. The urban population increased from 17.3 per cent in 1907 to 43.8 per cent in 1986 with nearly one-half of the population concentrated in greater Cairo and Alexandria. The total urban–rural population rates of growth indicate that the urban population multiplied at a faster pace than both the national and rural levels. The pace of urbanization shows a relative slowdown in the 1986 census as compared with the period before the 1976 census. The 1976 population census estimated that 1.4 million Egyptians were resident abroad.

According to the results of the 1986 population census, the number of Egyptians working or living in other Arab countries was officially estimated at 2.25 million. The government of Egypt believes that the current rate of population growth is too high, that it impedes development efforts, and frustrates the hopes for improving the quality of life for the Egyptians (CAPMAS, 1991).

## Ageing

According to 1986 census, the population below six years of age constitutes 19.2 per cent of the total population. The population below 12 years constitutes 34.1 per cent and the population from 12–64 years constitutes 63 per cent of the total population. However, those in the age group 65 years and above constitute only 2.9 per cent of the total population. Hence, the Egyptian population is considered a young population. Dependency ratio reached 37 per cent in the 1986 census.

Ageing is not yet considered a social or health problem in Egypt. However, the trend toward lower infant mortality indicates that in the near future ageing will be an emerging problem, and should therefore, currently be earmarked for strategic planning.

## CONCLUSION

Notwithstanding the untiring efforts of the various concerned ministries during the last few decades, nutrition problems—under- and over-nutrition—are still prevalent; at both ends of the spectrum. This necessitates more targeted efforts, with special emphasis on general education and nutrition education.

## REFERENCES

Abdel Ghany, S. A. (1986). Maternal nutrition and outcome of pregnancy. Ph.D. thesis. Faculty of Home Economics, Helwan University, 1986.

Abdou, I. A. (1965a). *Nutrition Status in the New Valley* (in Arabic). National Documentation Center, Dokki, Cairo, Egypt.

Abdou, I. A., Ali, H. E., and Lebshtein, A. K. (1965b). A study of the nutritional status of mothers, infants and young children, attending MCH centers in Cairo: I-The nutritional status of infants and young children. *Bulletin of Nutrition Institute*, **1**, 9–20.

Abdou, I. A., Ali, H. E., Said, A. K., Moussa, W. A., Demian, H. G., Soliman, A. M., and El-Hawary, L. H. (1967c). Incidence of nutritional deficiencies, goitre and dental caries among school children in Cairo. *Journal of the Egyptian Public Health Association*, **42**, 175–84.

Abdou, I. A., Farrag, F. M., and Guindi, A. F. (1968b). Prevalence of nutritional anaemia in the age group 6–18 years of rural, urban and industrial communities in Beheira governorate. *Bulletin of Nutrition Institute*, **4**, 81–106.

Abdou, I. A. and Mahfouz, A. (1967a). Heights and weights of school children in Cairo as indications of their nutritional status. *Journal of the Egyptian Public Health Association*, **42**, 114–24.

Abdou, I. A., and Mahfouz, A. (1968a). Comparative study of heights and weights of school children in different sectors of Cairo, other areas of UAR and foreign standards. *Bulletin of Nutrition Institute*, **4**, 53–68.

Abdou, I. A. and Moussa, W. A. (1975). Study of dietary factors causing growth retardation of boys in the Egyptian village. *Egyptian Journal of Nutrition*, **I**, 143.

Abdou, I. A., Shaker, M. S., Bishara, F. F., and El-Mogharbel, M. K. (1967b). A comparative study of the nutritional status of infants and pre-school children in different types of villages, urban sector and MCH centres of Beheira governorate. *Bulletin of Nutrition Institute*, **3**, 5–40.

Abdou, I. A., Shukry, A. S., Labib, F. M., and Moussa, W. A. (1975). Nitrogen balance studies on protein-rich food mixtures for pre-school children in Egypt. *Gazette of the Egyptian Pediatric Association*, **23**, 111–27.

Akre, J. (1989). Infant feeding; the physiological basis. *Bulletin of World Health Organization*. Supplement to Vol. 67.

Alderman, H. and Von Braun, J. (1984). The effect of the Egyptian food ration and subsidy system on income distribution and consumption. Research Report 45, International Food Policy Research Institute, Washington D.C..

Aly, H., *et al.* (1981). ARE National Food Consumption Study, Final Report, Nutrition Institute, Ministry of Health, Cairo

Aly, H. E., Moussa, W. A., Demian, H. G., Hasanyn, S. A., and Said, A. K. (1980). Anthropometric measurements of Cairo school children: A follow-up study. *Journal of the Egyptian Public Health Association*, **55**, 143–65.

Aly, H. E., Moussa, W. A., Said, A. K., and Ghoneim, F. M. (1981). Effect of food aid on nutritional status of beneficiaries in land reclamation projects. *Ain Shams Med. J.*, **32**, 205–14.

Aly, H. E., Said, A. K. Shaheen, F. M., Moussa, W. A., and Dongol, I. E. (1976). Evaluation of school lunch program at technical secondary schools of ARE. 1-Effect on height, weight and clinical picture. *Bulletin of Nutrition Institute*, **6**, 1–16.

Aly, H. E., Moussa, W. A., Maksoud, A. A., and Gharib, N. (1976). Effect of supplementary feeding on health and growth of infants and young children of low socioeconomic group in Egypt. *Bulletin of Nutrition Institution*, **6**, 37–59.

ARE (1978). Nutrition Status Survey. Aly, H. E., Dakroury, A., Said, K., Hussein, M. A., Ghoneim, F., Shaheen, F., *et al.* Final Report. MOH. CDC. USAID.

Calloway, D. H., Murphy, S. P., and Beaton, G. H. (1988). Food intake and human function. A Cross Project Perspective of Collaborative Research Support Program in Egypt, Kenya and Mexico. University of California, Berkeley.

Central Agency for Population Mobilization And Statistics (CAPMAS), 1991, Statistical Year Book, Cairo.

El-Molla, M. A. (1990). 'Glycosuria'. In: Ibrahim, Amal S. (ed). The Final Report of HES–HEP. Cairo.

FAO (1985). The Fifth World Food Survey. Food and Agriculture Organization of the United Nations, Rome.

FAO/UNICEF/WHO (1976). Methodology of nutritional surveillance. Technical Report Series 593, World Health Organization, Geneva.

FAO/WHO (1990). Meeting the Nutrition Challenge. A joint FAO/WHO Framework paper.

FAO/WHO/UNU (1985). Expert consultation, energy and protein requirements. *Technical Report Series 724*. World Health Organization, Geneva.

Galal, O. *et al.* (1987). The Collaborative Research Support Program (CRSP) on Food Intake and Human Function. Final Report Grant No. Dan - 1309-G-SS-1070-00. U.S. AID, Washington, D.C. 1987.

Girgis, S. M. (1987). Effect of long-term lactation on maternal health. Ph.D. thesis. Faculty of Home Economics, Helwan University, Helwan, Egypt.

Habib, N. (1987). Teenage obesity among preparatory schools in Ismailia. M.Sc. thesis, Suez Canal University.

Hussein, M. A., Hassan, H. A., Abdel-Ghaffar, A. A., and Salem, S. (1988). Effect of iron supplements on occurrence of diarrhoea among children in rural Egypt. *Food and Nutrition Bulletin*, **10**, 35–9.

Hussein, M. A. (1989). The effect of increasing food cost on the behavior of families towards feeding their members. Final Report. Nutrition Institute/Catholic Relief Services, Egypt, Cairo.

Hussein, M. A., Hassan, H. A., Noor, E. F., and El-Shafie, M. (1989). Nutritional assessment of pre-school children in Egypt. *Gazette of the Egyptian Pediatrics Association*, **37**, 27–35.

Hussein, M. A. Moussa, W. A., and El-Nahry, F. I. (1991). Community based low-cost weaning foods suitable for feeding infants and young children in Egypt within a package of PHC services. Nutrition Institute, Cairo, Egypt.

Moussa, W. A. (1973). Development of protein-rich food mixtures suitable for feeding infants and young children. M.D. thesis, Faculty of Medicine, Cairo University, Cairo.

Moussa, W. A. (1986). Dietary Assessment. Proceedings of the Intercountry Workshop on Nutrition Assessment, FAO/UN/Nutrition Institute, MOH, Cairo.

Moussa, W. A. (1987). Health Profile of Egypt. The Health Interview Survey: Final Report, Dietary Habits Publication No. 36/5. ARE Ministry of Health.

Moussa, W. A. (1988). Food Sources of Energy Proceedings of the CRSP Policy Workshop, Nutrition Institute, Cairo, Egypt.

Moussa, W. A. (1988a). Nutritional Status in Egypt. Health Profile of Egypt, Health Examination Survey. Final Report. Publication No. 38/1.

Moussa, W. A. (1989). Weights, heights and growth patterns in Egypt. Final Report of the Health Examination Survey (HES) of the Health Profile of Egypt (HPE) Publication No 38/2, December, 1988.

Moussa, W. A. (1990). Weaning foods. Proceedings of the International Conference on Food for Special Dietary and Medicinal Uses, Cairo, Egypt, *Bulletin of Nutrition Institute*. ARE. Special issue, 19–22.

Moussa, W. A., Aly, H. E. Goma, H. Mikhael, K. G., and Said, A. K. (1983). The role of infection in causation of malnutrition in urban areas of Egypt with special reference to diarrhoeal disease. *Urban Health Policy*, 44–7.

Moussa, W. A., Hegazy, M. E., Weber, C. (1988). Energy and protein bioavailability of toddlers. Diets in Rural Egyptian Community. Proceedings of 'Bioavailability 88', Norwich, U.K.

Moussa, W. A., Hegazy, M. E., Weber, C. (1989). Energy and protein bioavailability of Egyptian rural pre-schooler diets: Implication and application. *Proceedings of the 14th International Congress of Nutrition*, August 20–25, Seoul, Korea, 384.

Moussa, W. A., Sobhy, A. H., Mikhael, K. G., Hassan, T. M. and Aly, H. E. (1988a). Feeding and weaning practices of infants and children less than two years at Cairo governorate. *Bulletin of Nutrition Institute*, **8**, 82–100.

Moussa, W. A., Mikhael, K. G., Sobhy, A. H. and Aly, H. E. (1988b). Major determinants of adequacy of supplements during the weaning period. *Bulletin of Nutrition Institute*, **8**, 102–29.

Noor, E., Kirksey, A., Wacks, T., Jeome, N., McCbe, G., Aly, H., Galal, and Harrison, G. (1991). Mother–toddler interaction and care giving behavior in an Egyptian semi rural village. Federation of American Societies For Experimental Biology, Atlanta, G.A.

Oldham, L., Sholkami, H., Hadidi, H., and Wahba, S. (1990). Sociocultural factors influencing the prevalence of diarrhoeal disease in rural Upper Egypt. An ethnographic study of six villages, UNICEF.

Pinstrup-Andesan, Per (1987). Food prices and the poor in developing countries. In: Gittinger, J. Price, Leslie, Janne, and Hoisington, Caroline (eds). *Food Policy. EDI Series in Economic Development.* The Johns Hopkins University Press, Baltimore and London, 283.

Rihan, Z. E. and Lebshtein, A. K. (1971). Control of diabetes in different socio-economic groups. *Journal of the Egyptian Public Health Association*, **46**, 265–72.

Said, A. K. (1987). Personal habits, health status and medical care, Final Report, HIS, Health Profile of Egypt. Publication N 36/3.

Said, A. K., Moussa, W. A., Demian, H. G., Aref, N. M., and Aly, H. E., (1980). Follow-up study of nutritional deficiencies among Cairo school children. *Journal of the Egyptian Public Health Association*, **45**, 225–63.

Sarhan, A. A. (1982). Prevalence of obesity among preparatory school children in Cairo. M.S. thesis submitted to the High Institute of Public Health, University of Alexandria, Egypt.

Sayed, H. A., Osman, M. I., El-Zanaty, F. and Way, A. A., (1989). Egypt Demographic and Health Survey (DHS) 1988. Egypt National Population Council, Cairo, Egypt and Institute for Resource Development/Macro Systems Inc., Columbia, Maryland, USA.

Sherif, M. and Ibrahim, A. S. (1987). *The Profile of Cancer in Egypt.* The National Cancer Institute, Cairo.

Shukry, A. S., Barakat, M. R., El-Gammal R., and Kamel, L. M. (1972). An epidemiological study of protein–calorie malnutrition among rural population in Egypt. *Gaz Egypt-Ped Assc* , **20**, 151–67.

Tomkins, A. and Watson, F. (1989). Malnutrition and infection: A review. United Nations ACC/SCN.

WHO (1968). Nutritional anaemias. Report of a WHO Scientific Group. WHO Technical Report Series No 405, Geneva.

WHO (1974). Human Nutrition Requirements. WHO/EMRO Technical Report Series No. 61, Geneva.

WHO (1990). Diet, nutrition and the prevention of chronic diseases. Technical Report Series 797, Geneva.

WHO (1989). Guidelines for the Development of A Food and Nutrition Surveillance System for Countries in the Eastern Mediterranean Region. WHO/EMRO, Technical Publication No. 13, Geneva.

# Index

# SOCIAL SCIENCE LIBRARY

Oxford University Library Services
Manor Road
Oxford OX1 3UQ
Tel: (2)71093 (enquiries and renewals)
http://www.ssl.ox.ac.uk

## This is a NORMAL LOAN item.

We will email you a reminder before this item is due.

Please see http://www.ssl.ox.ac.uk/lending.html
for details on

- loan policies; these are also displayed on the
  notice boards and in our library guide.

- how to check when your books are due back.

- how to renew your books, including information
  on the maximum number of renewals.
  Items may be renewed if not reserved by
  another reader. Items must be renewed before
  the library closes on the due date.

- level of fines; fines are charged on overdue books.

Please note that this item may be recalled during Term.